A MARKETER'S GUIDE TO MEASURING ROI

TOOLS TO TRACK THE RETURNS FROM HEALTHCARE MARKETING EFFORTS

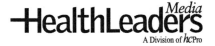

HealthLeaders *Media*
A Division of *hc*Pro

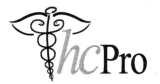

*hc*Pro

DAVID MARLOWE

David Marlowe, Author

Gienna Shaw, Editor

Michele Wilson, Executive Editor

Matthew Cann, Group Publisher

Jackie Diehl Singer, Graphic Artist

Doug Ponte, Cover Designer

Matthew Kuhrt, Copyeditor

Sada Preisch, Proofreader

Darren Kelly, Books Production Supervisor

Susan Darbyshire, Art Director

Claire Cloutier, Production Manager

Jean St. Pierre, Director of Operations

Advice given is general. Readers should consult professional counsel for specific legal, ethical, or clinical questions.

Arrangements can be made for quantity discounts. For more information, contact:

HCPro, Inc.
P.O. Box 1168
Marblehead, MA 01945
Telephone: 800/650-6787 or 781/639-1872
Fax: 781/639-2982
E-mail: *customerservice@hcpro.com*

HCPro, Inc. is the parent company of Healthleaders Media.
Visit HCPro at its World Wide Web sites:
www.healthleadersmedia.com, www.hcpro.com, and *www.hcmarketplace.com*

Contents

       A Marketer's Guide to Measuring ROI

Acknowledgments

This is the third book I have been involved with as an author or coauthor, and it never gets any simpler. Without support, advice, and an occasional good-natured push from friends, colleagues, and family this just can't be done.

First, I want to thank the folks at HealthLeaders Media for seeing the promise of this topic and for giving me the chance to put pen to paper (okay, fingers to keys, but you get the idea). In particular I want to thank Gienna Shaw and Michele Wilson and the rest of the staff at HealthLeaders Media. Gienna had the less-than-enviable job of working with me as the editor for the project. I think we set a record for the number of deadlines missed (all my fault), and she was always there to provide guidance and the requisite push to get back to work.

I also want to thank the many hospital-based and consulting-based colleagues who answered my call for potential ROI case studies. They gave their time to talk with me, review drafts, etc., without any return except the knowledge that they were sharing their expertise with their colleagues in the field. For a variety of reasons I could not include all of their case studies but I very much appreciate the help of everyone who came forward with information and support. While we have a long way to go in healthcare marketing before ROI tracking becomes a routine part of the process, there is a lot of impressive work going on out there.

My thanks go to the all of my clients and to the hundreds of people who have attended my ROI-related presentations over the past few years. Every time I do one of these projects or make a presentation on the topic I learn more and I hopefully get a bit better at the process.

Thank you to my friends in the healthcare marketing field who have supported me over the years and who encouraged me to dive into the authorship pool one more time. One of the best parts of being in this field is the friendships made and nurtured over a 30-year (and more to go) career.

Thank you to the leadership and staff of the Society for Healthcare Strategy and Market Development of the American Hospital Association. They saw the promise of this topic and agreed to work with HealthLeaders in marketing the book to healthcare marketing professionals. I've been very fortunate to be part of this organization for the past 27 years and on its Board for the past seven.

And then there is my family. A simple "thank you" really isn't enough here, but I'll give it my best shot. To my son, Daniel, who constantly reminds me of the joy and challenges of seeing the world through younger eyes. To my parents, who are always proud of what I have accomplished but still aren't quite sure of what I do for a living. And to my wife, Cathy, who has probably spent the equivalent of two years waiting for me to "just finish this page." I love all of you very much.

About the author

As the principal of Strategic Marketing Concepts, a healthcare marketing consulting firm based in Ellicott City, MD, **David Marlowe** helps hospitals and health systems develop strategic marketing plans, conduct market research and marketing function assessments, create medical staff marketing, develop new programs, set pricing strategies, and deal with healthcare delivery system marketing issues. Prior to forming Strategic Marketing Concepts, Marlowe served as vice president of strategic consulting for First Strategic Group in Whittier, CA; vice president of strategic services for Market Strategies, Inc., in Richmond, VA; vice president of planning and marketing for St. Agnes Hospital in Baltimore; and director of marketing for Harbor Health System in Baltimore.

Marlowe has more than 27 years of healthcare marketing and planning experience as a consultant and a provider-based executive. In addition, he has held adjunct faculty positions at Avila College in Kansas City, MO, and the University of Baltimore. He is a frequent author and lecturer for national and local professional organizations such as the American College of Healthcare Executives, the Forum for Healthcare Strategists, the Medical Group Management Association, and the Society for Healthcare Strategy and Market Development (SHSMD). Marlowe, the 2007 president-elect of SHSMD, was honored in 2005 by the organization, which gave him the Award for Individual Professional Excellence, the highest honor bestowed by this national professional association.

He is the coauthor and editor of the book *Building a Foundation for Effective Healthcare Market Research*, the author of the book *Healthcare Marketing Plans That Work*, and he serves on the editorial board of various healthcare marketing publications.

Marlowe holds a BS degree in accounting from Syracuse University and a Masters of Management degree in marketing from the J. L. Kellogg Graduate School of Management at Northwestern University.

A Marketer's Guide to Measuring ROI

Introduction

The concept of measuring a return on investment (ROI) from marketing—or, simply put, what we are getting in return for the organizational resources we spend on marketing efforts—is not really all that new. When I came out of graduate school in 1980, flush with the training that comes from a classical marketing degree and definitely full of a fair degree of naiveté, I attempted to measure the impact of a marketing promotional effort on volumes coming into the hospital I was working for. Unfortunately, we had no way to connect marketing efforts to patient volumes, no way to track patient revenues, and no way to get a handle on the costs of services sold (all concepts that we'll discuss in more detail later on in this book). As you can imagine, that effort was a spectacular failure.

So I gave up trying to measure ROI in detail and focused instead on developing marketing plan objectives that could at least be reasonably supported by the data and information systems available to us in provider settings. By the mid-1990s, however, the world had changed and I started talking more about tracking ROI as a concept at professional educational programs. In the late 1990s I had a chance to work with a client on the tracking of hard ROI from a very focused marketing effort. ("Hard" ROI simply means that the results are measured by the actual collected revenues after taking into account the actual cost of the effort.)

Over time, more of these opportunities have come along and the term ROI has shown up much more prominently in healthcare marketing literature and in educational programs at the local and national level. By 2006, I was speaking to audiences almost monthly about tracking ROI for healthcare marketing and finally, in early 2007, I was asked by the folks at HealthLeaders Media (a division of the Marblehead, MA–based HCPro, Inc., publishing company) to turn the concept into a book.

Along the way I have learned a lot about both the need for ROI tracking and the challenges in implementing such an effort. Here are some key axioms of ROI analysis for healthcare marketers gleaned from this personal learning curve:

- ROI is very challenging to implement (we'll discuss the reasons why later in the book).

- Despite the challenges, the nature of our industry is making it increasingly essential that all provider-based marketing efforts try to implement some degree of ROI analysis.

- A lot of what we do in the healthcare marketing sector is not designed to immediately drive volumes and financial returns. As a result, these activities are not candidates for ROI tracking. But that doesn't relieve provider-based marketers from the responsibility for establishing other quantifiable metrics.

- You should start small when it comes to ROI tracking efforts. Gain experience through one relatively simple tracking process and then expand the portfolio.

 A Marketer's Guide to Measuring ROI

What you need to know about ROI

While this book provides what I hope are helpful guidelines for the development and implementation of ROI tracking efforts, there are no absolute rules. Whatever the organization's leadership is willing to accept in the way of assumptions is okay—at least for that organization. That having been said, there are a few more important things to remember about ROI as you read through this book:

- ROI means that there is a financial return. If no revenue was generated as a result of the marketing effort, there is no ROI. Media coverage, image, participation, and goodwill are all important outcomes, but they are not measurable by an ROI analysis.

- Hard effort ROI means that the measurement takes into account all aspects of the financial side of measurement. This includes revenues net of contractual allowances and bad debts (collected revenues), and revenues net of "costs of services sold" or direct variable costs.

- Finally, it is absolutely crucial that you determine and put in place the tracking systems and key assumptions up front—before the marketing effort begins.

Why are we putting so much emphasis on ROI for healthcare marketing and indeed on tracking the impact of marketing in healthcare in general? Marketing in the healthcare field is about 25–30 years old, depending on whom you ask and how you define marketing. While there has always been an interest in measuring the results of marketing for provider organizations, the level of interest has gone up radically in recent years. This is being fueled by increasing financial pressures on providers and, in turn, increasing pressures to show that all elements of the management arena are delivering value for the resources used. Marketing can no longer use the excuse that it is too new to be subjected to measurement. Leaders are looking for measurable results—and effort ROI is about as definitive as those results can get.

The balance of this book will look at the definition of effort ROI and how that concept exists outside of the healthcare field. We will then spend a fair amount of time looking at the factors that make ROI measurement challenging in the provider arena, what logistics have to be faced to measure effort ROI, and how effort ROI is actually implemented. We will also look at metrics other than ROI (and when they might be more appropriate), the impact of ROI on the overall marketing budget, and what to consider in terms of services to use for a first ROI tracking effort.

Test your understanding of hard ROI

Before we get started, however, let's warm up with a quiz to get you thinking about what exactly goes into a rigorous examination of ROI for marketing activities. Read the following three examples. Which, if any, is likely to allow the organization to measure the hard ROI from the marketing effort?

Case A

Community General Hospital hires an external public relations firm to support a more aggressive effort to capture media placements and public

A Marketer's Guide to Measuring ROI

visibility in its market. The firm works closely with hospital staff and achieves the target goal of eight media placements (print, radio, etc.) per month. The cost of the effort is $65,000, the bulk of which is spent on agency fees. A summary report, developed by the agency, shows that over a specific period of time the effort resulted in coverage that would have cost $142,000 if the hospital had purchased equivalent media space (column inches, radio minutes, etc.).

Case B

Memorial Medical Center (MMC) conducts a regular series of health screenings in its service area. During the fiscal year, MMC screened 8,500 people. Of this group, 440 were found to have a health condition that warranted a referral to a physician and/or a specific healthcare service. MMC followed up by scheduling appointments and giving referrals to these people. MMC could also track individual participants who later used hospital services or made appointments with employed physicians. The hospital used predetermined criteria to identify referrals who were new patients.

Patients who went through the screenings and received follow-up care generated $643,500 in collected revenues over the next nine months. The cost of the health fair was $119,250.

Case C

St. Mary's Hospital has a cardiology preference share in its primary service area of 35%. For two years, the organization works to upgrade its capabilities in this area. It develops a brand new cardiac catheterization lab, recruits two cardiologists and a cardiac surgeon, and develops a state-of-the-art cardiac rehab center as part of its fitness facility. St. Mary's develops and launches a

nine-month promotional and advertising campaign that costs $450,000.
Eighteen months after the launch of the campaign, St. Mary's 35%
cardiology preference share increases to 48%.

So what's the right answer?

Cases A and C illustrate solid examples of quantifiable measurements of
marketing activities, but they are not real ROI analyses. Only the second
example, Case B, contains the elements needed to measure a true return on
investment for a healthcare marketing effort. After reading this book, you'll
understand why.

A Marketer's Guide to Measuring ROI

What is ROI?

What is ROI?

The traditional accounting-textbook definition of return on investment (ROI) is net income after expenses divided by owner's equity. As a mathematical equation, it would look like this:

$$\text{ROI} = \frac{\text{Net income} - \text{expenses}}{\text{Owner's equity}}$$

Owner's equity is the amount of the business "owned" by the owners or stockholders and not owed to third parties. In other words, owner's equity is assets minus liabilities.

For example, Company Q has a net income (income after expenses) of $500,000 and an owner's equity of $18.3 million. If you divide the net income by the owner's equity, the ROI is .027, or 2.7%.

What's the right ROI?

At this point, you might be wondering what percent constitutes a good ROI. There is no magic number. Rather, the answer depends upon the industry norms for companies similar to this one and its owners' other investment opportunities. In some industries, a 2.7% ROI might be considered an excellent return—time to celebrate a good year. In others, a 2.7% ROI would indicate that it is time for the board of directors to fire the senior management team and bring in a turnaround group. If a company has assets that are fairly liquid, its owner or owners might opt to get out of the business and pursue options that offer higher returns. On the other hand, if the nature of the company's industry is such that liquidating the assets would likely result in a significant loss, then the practicality of pursuing a higher ROI may be limited.

What is effort ROI?

That's the traditional definition of ROI, appropriate for an entire organization's finances. For our purposes, however, we need to get more focused. So we'll use an approach called "effort" ROI. That's the revenue (net of costs) that comes from a specific marketing endeavor. Effort ROI allows us to measure how much income we generated from marketing activities such as:

- A $250,000 media advertising campaign that targeted adults age 50 and older for joint replacement surgery

A Marketer's Guide to Measuring ROI

- A $150,000 direct-mail campaign aimed at driving consumers to a cardiac-related health screening tool on a hospital Web site

- A $400,000 outlay to promote and implement an extensive series of health screening efforts among key audiences

- A $30,000 investment to expand hours of operation for a freestanding diagnostic imaging center to allow more convenient consumer access

- $65,000 to add a physician representative to reach potential referring physicians in a tertiary service area

The formula for effort ROI is net revenue after marketing expenses times 100 divided by the cost of the marketing effort. The mathematical equation would look like this:

$$\text{Effort ROI} = \frac{\text{Net revenue} - \text{marketing expenses}}{\text{Marketing expenses}} \times 100$$

Net revenue, in this case, is the revenue collected from patients determined to have come from the specific marketing effort less a factor for "costs of services sold."

How is effort ROI used outside of healthcare?

I think it is safe to say that there is a much more ingrained organizational focus on tracking the impact of marketing and overall effort ROI in the traditional for-profit corporate world than in the healthcare provider sector. For a much more detailed overview of the role of effort ROI tracking outside of healthcare, I refer the reader to a book written by James Lenskold called *Marketing ROI: The Path to Campaign, Customer and Corporate Profitability* (American Marketing Association, 2003).

Lenskold's book provides a very detailed view of the challenges and processes required to measure ROI from marketing efforts, but it also indirectly provides some very striking contrasts to the world of hospital and health-system marketing:

- None of the examples in the book relate to healthcare and/or the non-profit world. All are based in the core Fortune 1000 world of industrial services, consumer products, etc. This is by no means meant to be a criticism of the Lenskold book, but rather a striking portrait of how this concept is just not even associated with the healthcare provider field.

- Clearly reflecting the intended audience, the book states that "[T]he ultimate purpose of marketing is to generate profitable sales, and it is to the benefit of shareholders, executives, and marketers to manage the budget as an investment." For a Fortune 1000 firm I couldn't agree more. And certainly there is a profit/positive financial return motive in

A Marketer's Guide to Measuring ROI

the healthcare provider sector. But we also have other imperatives that are not immediately financially driven, and thus may mitigate the need for marketing always to have an ROI end (or at least a financial ROI).

- The Lenskold book also quotes a study by a third party conducted among marketing executives in the United States and the United Kingdom. In this study, 68% of the participants noted that ROI tracking for marketing efforts was "very difficult" to achieve. I provide this information so as to give the reader some modest degree of comfort that the healthcare marketing world is perhaps not so far behind our counterparts in other fields.

It's not unusual for firms in other industries (especially the consumer product world) to set target or threshold ROI goals for various marketing initiatives. In other words, the organization won't implement a specific marketing effort unless it has a very good chance of achieving an ROI of at least a certain percentage. Of course, taking this position indicates that the organization or the industry that the organization is in has a good track record of knowing the usual and customary ROI for different marketing approaches.

But the healthcare industry really doesn't have any standard measure for the typical ROI on specific efforts. Perhaps the closest parallel we have is a set of general guidelines for determining which service lines will get priority on marketing resources based on their margins of return. For example, there is a general consensus that orthopedic surgery has a relatively high margin, whereas obstetrics often barely breaks even or even loses money. Of course this is not universal—there are hospitals that report positive margins for obstetrical care and thus are willing to market that service actively.

Contribution margin—revenues after variable expenses—is often not the only consideration when it comes to deciding where to put marketing resources. Competitive factors, organizational mission, and even politics can also play a role. For example:

- Mercy Hospital's obstetrical service has experienced declining volumes for a number of years, primarily driven by changes in local demographics. In addition, obstetrical care shows a loss (prior to contribution to overhead) of more than $2,000 per case. Looking at this from a business standpoint only, no marketing investment should be made in obstetrical care. However, obstetrics service is a key element in the religious mission of this provider. As a result, the hospital decides to develop an extensive and fairly costly promotional campaign aimed at driving preference and potential usage of Mercy for deliveries.

- Pulmonary admissions show a positive margin for County General, but that margin ranks about 18th out of 25 possible service lines. The lead pulmonary group, however, is part of a multispecialty group practice that contributes close to half of all the admissions coming to County General. In addition, one member of the pulmonary group is on the board and another is the incoming elected president of the medical staff. This puts a great deal of pressure on the hospital to market pulmonary health issues and services.

A Marketer's Guide to Measuring ROI

An example of effort ROI

Let's go back to looking at effort ROI outside of the healthcare provider sector. The following example clearly demonstrates the measurable return on investment for a specific, easy-to-define marketing activity. Although the case is older (and the numbers somewhat outdated) it is still a useful example.

Three Lakes Amusement Park is open from April through October. Visitors pay one price for access to all rides and shows. They pay extra for parking, souvenirs, food, and arcade games. Weekends and weekdays between late June and the end of August are busiest. Business drops in early June and early September. Three Lakes distributes discount coupons at key locations in the business area that give 50% off or two admissions for the price of one. These coupons are good only during the park's slow periods. Management realizes that it has significant fixed costs that will occur whether the park is busy or not. So it makes sense to give a discount to attract customers during those slow periods, knowing they'll spend money on items that aren't covered by admission.

ROI analysis information and assumptions

Elements of the marketing effort:

- Distribution of discount coupons to key sites at a total cost of $21,000

Time period for tracking results:

- Coupon-driven volumes are counted on a daily basis, but the final ROI analysis is not performed until the end of the season

Tracking methodology:
- Very low-tech but nonetheless effective—the coupons turned in each target day are counted and recorded

Factor for business they would have gotten anyway:
- Based on survey research done each year, the Three Lakes management determined that 30% of the people using the discount coupons would have come to the park that day anyway

Results/revenues/costs of services provided:
- Over the course of the season, 14,500 people were admitted to the park using the discount coupons

- When the "business would have gotten anyway" factor was considered, the volume gained is 10,150 people

Revenues generated from these 10,150 people:
- Admissions = 10,150 x $14.00 (half off) = $142,100

- Parking = 2,538 x $6.00 = $15,228 (Note: experience shows four people come per car and no discount was given for parking)

- Other = 10,150 x $27.00 = $274,050 (Note: experience shows that each person coming to the park will spend another $27 on food, prizes, amusements, etc.)

A Marketer's Guide to Measuring ROI

- Direct cost of services sold = 35%

- Net revenues from customers "gained" from the marketing effort =
  $280,396 ($142,100 + $15,228 + $274,050 x 0.65)

Effort ROI calculation:

$$ROI = \frac{\text{Net revenue} - \text{marketing expenses}}{\text{Marketing expenses}} \times 100$$

$$ROI = \frac{(\$280,396 - \$21,000)}{\$21,000} \times 100$$

$$ROI \text{ percent} = 1{,}235\%$$

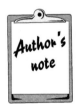

Author's note Clearly this is a very good marketing effort for Three Lakes and one they are likely to continue in future years.

What factors make effort ROI tracking more challenging for healthcare providers?

What factors make effort ROI tracking more challenging for healthcare providers?

Healthcare is different

A common theme among healthcare marketers is that healthcare does indeed differ from other sectors of the economy, and marketing in healthcare differs from the marketing in other areas. Many of the techniques used by marketers in other fields don't carry over readily to the marketing of healthcare services. We can't pay bonuses or incentives for referrals. We can't guarantee our work. We are limited in what we can do with pricing (so far). Quality is very hard to measure and there are, at this writing, no industry-wide standards. Packaging has little meaning. We have to be much more careful about what we say in our advertising. We have much stronger privacy restrictions that limit the usage of our own data.

In addition, healthcare has market structure factors that make the purchase process different from that of almost any other sector. No one fully understands healthcare pricing and reimbursement. Patients receive services from hospitals, but those services are usually ordered by an independent third party (the doctor) and paid for by yet another third party (the insurer), who in turn is often paid by yet one more party (the employer). Imagine getting your dry cleaning done that way! The decision process in the usage of health services is driven heavily by emotion, even if we make efforts to apply logic. And finally, we have by far the largest service sector in the country that no one wants to use. People want to buy cars, go to restaurants, stay at hotels, and shop for new clothes. Very few get a serious kick out of having surgery or getting an MRI.

This market structure differential factor carries over to the measurement of effort return on investment (ROI). Other industries definitely have their challenges in trying to measure effort ROI, but healthcare has some elements that are either unique or more pronounced. This chapter will look at some of those challenges and, where practical, some opportunities to deal with them. As you read this, I would ask you not to be too discouraged. The fact that we have industry-unique challenges doesn't make the process impossible. Recognizing the following ten challenges is half the battle in working around them.

Time delay in usage

The usage of healthcare services is rarely predictable in terms of which person will use a service at a specific point in time. We know that a certain number of people out of 1,000 will need a cardiac catheterization in the coming year, but we don't know *which* people. In addition, for most healthcare services there has to be a viable clinical need for care before services can be rendered and paid for. As a result, there are natural and system time delays between the time marketing may influence consideration of a service and actual usage of the service. For example:

    A Marketer's Guide to Measuring ROI

- Program developments and strong promotional efforts may convince a consumer that Hospital A is the market leader for cardiac care—but it could be years before that individual needs cardiac services.

- Relationship-building efforts aimed at referring physicians may convince them to use the specialists at Hospital B for a specific service, but before they can do so there have to be patients coming into the practice with that need. Those patients may also need to get approval from their health insurance carriers, which could delay usage further.

- The need for ER services could be three minutes, three weeks, three months, or three years after a marketing effort convinces an individual that the ER at Hospital C is the best choice.

- A marketing effort may convince a patient that Hospital D and its related surgeons are the best choice for bariatric surgery. But the patient must attend required classes, complete clinical tests, and undergo psychiatric evaluation before the surgery can be performed—and this takes 3–6 months to complete.

- And even the best marketers have to wait nine months for the results of any successful effort on behalf of obstetrical services.

There is no practical or ethical way to speed up the usage of most healthcare services. Part of the overall marketing process and the process associated with effort ROI tracking has to be the recognition that it takes time for service needs to develop, and thus you must allow time for appropriate tracking.

Author's note

Ability to plan for usage

As marketers, we need to recognize that healthcare services fall into different categories of "plan-ability" and thus react differently to marketing efforts. This, in turn, affects whether we can track effort ROI effectively.

There are three broad categories in the healthcare field when it comes to the ability of consumers and referring physicians to plan usage:

Emergency care. These are the true life-threatening situations where there is no planning involved and usage may come down to geographic proximity or emergency protocols as opposed to a careful consideration of image, capabilities, etc. Examples include heart attacks, stroke, major accidents, trauma, neurosurgery, etc.

Urgent care. These are clinical cases where care is needed soon but perhaps not in the next hour. Time is not plentiful, but planning is possible—and users/referrers can consider issues other than quick access. Examples include surgery on a knee for a sports injury, a colonoscopy driven by specific symptoms, removal of a skin cancer growth, etc.

Elective care. These are clinical cases where the care is mostly or totally optional, or where the care is needed but there are many places where it can be received in order to get results. Examples include plastic surgery, laser eye surgery, lab tests, imaging tests, etc.

Urgent and elective services lend themselves more to effort ROI tracking. Emergency care services can certainly be influenced by marketing, but the time frame to see results is usually longer.

Lack of timely information

This is perhaps the most significant challenge to the implementation of viable effort ROI tracking. Provider information systems are not often geared to give managers timely information related to volumes generated, revenues collected, or expenses incurred in the provision of care. Clearly, effort ROI tracking is not possible if we can't determine how much volume came in, the revenue generated, or the cost of services sold.

In the pursuit of case examples for this book, I frequently found situations where the necessary information is months behind the time period being measured, and/or the financial arm of the organization could not provide a viable estimate of the direct costs of providing services.

In fairness to provider information/financial systems and the staff who manage them, not all of the delays are internal. It is not unusual for insurance carriers to take months to settle on payment for specific cases. Until this occurs we don't know the revenues (net of contractual allowances) for the care. In addition, as healthcare costs shift more and more to consumers, we may encounter time delays in measuring revenue as we attempt to collect larger levels of deductibles and copays.

Before you start any effort ROI measurements, talk with the financial department to determine when they can provide financial results and whether they can provide a figure for direct costs or costs of services sold. If this last item is not readily available, most provider financial departments can develop such a percentage, but it may take them some time—and it may not be their highest priority in the face of other issues. Giving them 3–6 months of lead time is a better approach than asking for the figure a few days before the analysis is due.

Lack of marketing tracking systems

Many healthcare providers lack systems to connect a specific marketing effort directly to patient usage. Key identification information is not collected at events, seminars, from promotional inquiries, etc. Key questions are not asked or recorded at registration. There is no call center, or the function is decentralized. The Web structure is largely passive, with no interactive ability to register or get immediate responses.

As we will discuss later in this chapter, effort ROI can be done when there is no viable direct-tracking system in hand, but it makes things more challenging and perhaps a bit more reliant upon assumptions as to what marketing did or did not accomplish.

The development of inquiry and tracking systems is a key component of any marketing infrastructure. If these are not in place then perhaps the priority is on that effort over the tracking of ROI.

Marketing goals that aren't always aimed at driving volumes

Sometimes our marketing efforts are aimed primarily or exclusively at driving volumes and revenues to the organization. In those cases effort ROI is a viable measure that you should consider. But a lot of what we do in the healthcare marketing field is not immediately aimed at driving volume. Much is aimed at brand-building—driving awareness, preference, image, etc. Over time, these contribute to bringing in or retaining volumes, but this is secondary to the original purpose of the marketing effort. In these cases, effort ROI is not a viable metric—but you can plan for and put in place other metrics.

Some healthcare marketing can never be measured in terms of ROI

Almost every provider organization in the country—from university medical centers to local family practice offices—gets involved in small-scale, community-based events and sponsorships. This is a reality of life in marketing and public relations circles. Examples of these small-scale, community efforts include:

- A float in the annual Fourth of July parade

- A sponsorship sign on the outfield wall of the Little League ball park

- A half-page ad in the program guide for the local high school's spring musical

By and large these efforts are not aimed at generating volumes and revenues, so you should not measure them with effort ROI. The true "return" from these efforts is community visibility and goodwill.

Establish policies relating to the types and number of community event/sponsorship activities the organization will support, but don't expend any serious efforts trying to measure ROI for these small-scale community-relations activities.

Most healthcare marketers aren't experts in financial analysis

I make this point with a good degree of trepidation, because I don't want to come across as being critical of my fellow marketers. But the truth is that most of the professionals on the marketing/public relations side of the healthcare provider sector have limited training and background in financial analysis and systems, and effort ROI is very much a financially and statistically driven effort. Because of this, there can be reluctance on the part of marketers to attempt such an effort.

If it is any consolation to my colleagues, I probably wouldn't ask the financial managers to design our promotional materials, manage community outreach events, or set up sales processes—and most of them wouldn't want to, anyway.

While it isn't practical to go back and get a degree in accounting or finance, I highly encourage marketers to get more familiar with both general and healthcare-specific financial issues, such as net revenues, contribution margins, variable and fixed expenses, etc. And it is imperative to bring the financial staff into the effort ROI process early so that key assumptions can be agreed upon prior to any measurement attempts.

Marketers may claim too much as part of effort ROI

This is probably not a challenge that is unique to the healthcare provider industry, but it is still an issue that marketers must recognize. Unless your organization is totally new or the service being marketed is brand-new, the organization provided care and had volumes before the marketing efforts started. Effort ROI needs to focus on volumes and revenues gained. To claim anything more than that will severely undermine the credibility of the marketing function.

This may better be illustrated by example. The marketing/public relations department at Oceanside Regional Hospital is asked to market the services of the organization's sleep lab. Historically, the lab averages about 25 new cases a month, with some minor fluctuations. The marketing department launches the campaign, and over the next 90 days the sleep lab gets 150 total cases. In its post-campaign review, the head of the marketing department types up a report crediting the campaign for all 150 cases. The only problem with this claim is that, based on past performance, the sleep lab would likely have gotten 75 cases anyway. So although the head of the marketing department might be justified in claiming the additional 75 cases, he or she is wrong to claim the full 150.

I believe that few of the professionals in our field would ever do this deliberately, but it is possible to overcount returns through mistakes in analysis.

Marketing involves many elements, and ROI can only go so far

It isn't unusual for a marketing communications effort to involve multiple modalities. For example, a campaign focusing on driving consumer preference for and usage of orthopedic surgery might involve advertising (radio, television, and outdoor), events, hospital newsletters, and an e-mail blast. There is a sound reason that we take this approach—our aim is to use the confluence of all of these communications vehicles to reinforce each other and to create an impression on the desired audience. Someone hears the radio spot (multiple times), sees the television ad, drives past the billboard a few times, and reads the newsletter article. Taken all together, the message motivates the person to contact the organization to pursue care for an orthopedic issue that has bothered him or her for a while.

With good planning and solid analytical work we may well be able to measure the effort ROI on the entire orthopedic marketing effort—the $300,000 spent on the six-month campaign. But the chances of measuring the ROI for the radio spots versus the outdoor billboards versus the newsletter articles are fairly slim—and it may not be worth the effort anyway. Unless each communications source has its own call-to-action channel (such as a different inquiry phone number for each source), the only viable way to measure which source drove individuals to act is to ask them. While this certainly can and should be done in order to examine the effectiveness of specific media, experience shows that consumer recall of specific sources is spotty at best.

Let me illustrate this last point by an example. In the mid-1980s many hospitals started physician referral programs. Most of these programs were supported by computer software programs, and these programs contained a field prompting the staff to ask how people heard about the program. One of the more commonly noted sources was the yellow pages in the local phone book. As a result, the organization ramped up its phone-book advertisements.

They spent more money on bigger, more colorful ads. Within a year or two, however, the industry discovered that consumers *really* learned about the referral programs from other media advertising and from family, friends, and coworkers. They only went to the yellow pages to get the phone number when they were already ready to call. Patients had vastly overstated the role that the yellow pages played in their decision-making process—and soon the size of the advertising and the related expenditures declined significantly.

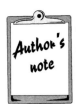 At least in the beginning, focus effort ROI measurements on the total campaign rather than on individual campaign elements.

Leaders may have unrealistic expectations and a lack of patience

This challenge certainly is not unique to healthcare but we do seem to have our fair share of it. There is a strong focus among healthcare leaders on the financial situation in the current fiscal year. As a result, they often look for immediate results from marketing and business-development efforts. In this "what have you done for me lately?" approach, executive leaders look for returns in the current quarter or (if we are lucky) the current fiscal year.

In these types of cases, ROI becomes return on expenditure, or ROE, a term that is not readily found in financial or accounting circles. As noted above, usage of healthcare is something that takes time to develop. Marketing efforts truly are investments that can take a while to bear fruit—often well beyond the current fiscal year.

As we'll discuss later in the book, it is essential that the organization's leadership agree on a reasonable time period for the measurement of effort ROI. Marketers must emphasize that, with limited exceptions, marketing efforts take time to develop returns, and that healthcare usage does not fit easily into fiscal year parameters.

What must we have in place to conduct an effort ROI analysis for a healthcare marketing activity?

What must we have in place to conduct an effort ROI analysis for a healthcare marketing activity?

Seven steps to effort ROI

This chapter will walk the reader through the process of measuring effort return on investment (ROI) for healthcare marketing. While it has been noted before, it is definitely worth noting again: The tracking mechanisms and the key assumptions discussed here must be in place and agreed upon *before* the marketing effort starts.

Step 1: Define the program or service being marketed

The very first step in the effort ROI process is to ensure that everyone agrees as to the scope of the program or clinical service that received the marketing support. This might sound almost silly—don't we know what program we were marketing? You'd think so, but I've had ROI project engagements where the individuals involved in the work didn't initially agree on whether the marketing was for MRI or all diagnostic imaging, or if it was for the surgery center or only for orthopedic surgery.

Before diving too far into the work of measuring effort ROI, make sure everyone agrees on the parameters of the services or program covered.

Step 2: Get consensus on direct, indirect, and noncredited returns

One of the key up-front assumptions that requires clear consensus before the measurement of effort ROI begins is what returns to accept as coming from the marketing effort in question. As noted earlier, there is no absolute rule here. Whatever is acceptable to the leadership of the organization works—and that might vary from organization to organization. Some examples might help to illustrate this point:

- Central State Hospital (CSH) develops a physician liaison program, something the organization has never had before. After the initial year of work, the effort of the physician liaison is shifted to target primary care physicians in a secondary market. These physicians currently send little or no volume to CSH. Any volume over historical levels coming to CSH from these doctors in the year after the refocusing of the liaison's work is credited to the marketing/business-development effort with no clinical service restrictions.

- Sunnyside Hospital owns a freestanding endoscopy suite as a joint venture with a group of gastroenterologists. The hospital conducts a targeted direct-mail effort to promote endoscopies and colonoscopies in appropriate circumstances. The effort is tracked by the use of a dedicated phone line and by information requested of the patients during registration. Direct credited returns from the promotion include any gastroenterology-related services. Indirect credited returns include any colon-rectal surgery care. A few individuals who received the mailing received care at Sunnyside for heart, neurological, orthopedic, and other non-GI related care during the measurement period. The hospital leadership opts not to credit these volumes to the direct-mail effort.

- Mid-Suburban Hospital conducts a regular series of classes for women who have never had a child but are considering getting pregnant. These "First-Time Mom" programs are promoted via a number of channels. Participant information is collected at registration and is compared with patient utilization information later to do a reconciliation of marketing efforts to actual volumes. For example:

    Ms. Smith attends the class and a year later delivers a child at Mid-Suburban. Her activity is considered a direct return from the OB-related marketing effort.

    Ms. Jones attends the class and six months later has GYN surgery at Mid-Suburban. Her volume is considered an indirect return, but is credited to the marketing effort.

    Ms. West attends the class and four months later has surgery on her knee because she injured it participating in a 5K race. While she was influenced by the OB-related marketing effort and has no history of using Mid-Suburban, her volume is considered noncredited and is not counted as a return coming from the marketing effort (per the Mid-Suburban leadership).

Whenever I present the Mid-Suburban example to a live audience, all of the participants agree that Ms. Smith should be counted as a return coming from the marketing effort. Usually a bit more than half feel that Ms. Jones should also be counted, although some say that it is a stretch. When it comes to Ms. West, however, only about a quarter feel that her volume should be counted. My response to this is that while the conservative approach is to count only the women who, like Ms. Smith, deliver a child at the hospital, any of the returns could be considered if the leadership is amenable to doing so. This is clearly one of the assumptions that must be agreed upon up front, however.

Step 3: Measure the cost of the marketing effort

A key component in the measurement of effort ROI from marketing is a clear understanding of the marketing expenditures. Elements that go into this component include:

- The cost of designing promotional-related materials (e.g., advertising creative fees, graphic design costs).

- The costs of any media advertising placements (e.g., print ads, radio time, outdoor boards, direct-mail postage and handling).

- The costs associated with any events, programs, or educational sessions (e.g., invitations, space, audio-visual, promotional items).

- Allocated support activity costs—costs associated with marketing support work generated by the specific marketing effort. For example, let's assume that Hospital P outsources its call center to a third-party firm

A Marketer's Guide to Measuring ROI

and pays an average of $7.50 per call to that firm. A specific marketing effort generates 3,300 calls during the measurement period. As a result, a cost of $24,750 ($7.50 x 3,300) should be included in the marketing costs.

- Allocated internal staff time from marketing, public relations, and other areas. For example, a specific marketing effort by the Southside Multi-Specialty Medical Group required approximately 125 staff hours to implement. Since this was spread out over a few staff people, the simplest and fairest approach is to take an average hourly rate (say $25) and multiply that number by the estimated staff time. In this case the cost would be $3,125.

 Some organizations consider marketing/public relations staff time as a given and not part of any specific marketing effort. As a result, that cost is not included in effort ROI measurements. I believe in a more conservative approach—that staff time would have been used for other efforts if it wasn't taken up by the effort being measured. Including allocated staff costs is more appropriate and will improve the credibility of the measurement. But remember, a reasonable estimate will do.

Step 4: Track returns from the marketing effort

This is perhaps the hardest part of the overall effort ROI work. How do we connect marketing effort A to patient usage B? In an ideal setting there is a mechanism in place to clearly connect the two and to show that the patient came to us as a result of the marketing effort. Some examples could include:

- **Paper or electronic coupons.** Coupons probably have very limited utility in a healthcare setting, but this low-tech approach still works as a way to connect a marketing effort directly to specific usage. A coupon giving the holder a discount on a screening test of some kind (e.g., mammography) would illustrate this point.

- **A coupon-like mechanism.** An example here is a freestanding breast health center or a physical therapy center that distributes "prescription pads" with information about the program, driving directions, etc. People bringing in these "prescriptions" or referrals for service clearly connect the usage to the specific physicians who were involved in the marketing effort.

- **A unique phone number.** The organization creates a unique phone number for the promotional effort. This works best if the effort is going to go on for a while (two years or more).

- **A unique identifier number.** A direct-mail campaign has a unique number printed on each item. Individuals receiving this mailing can use that number to register for an online screening test. If they show up as a patient for that clinical area during a predetermined number of months, their information can be compared to the people who took the online test.

- **Patient identification.** Information about the individual (e.g., name, address, phone number, age) is collected as part of the marketing process. This might occur at an event or online. This information can

 A Marketer's Guide to Measuring ROI

then be compared to patient information to see if patients used the clinical service related to the promotion.

- **Questions at registration.** Registration staff can ask questions related to how people heard about the service, if they attended a specific event, who their referring physician is, etc.

 On the surface, asking patients a question about marketing sources at registration seems to be the optimal tracking mechanism. But healthcare marketers almost universally find this doesn't work. While consumer recall of the source of the information can often be faulty, the primary problem is the lack of consistency in implementing the registration questions by the registration staff. If a computerized registration system is used, this information is usually part of an optional field and the system will not stop the registration staff if they opt to skip the question. Or, under pressure to handle a large volume of patients, registration staff members skip optional questions for the sake of speed. Registration tracking only appears to work when there is careful training, significant oversight, and appropriate incentives to supervisors and staff to make sure they ask the appropriate questions.

Frequently, however, the ideal situation does not exist. The organization does not have a call center, or cannot ensure reliable responsiveness from registration staff. In those cases we need to consider whether the volumes have moved an appreciable degree from historical activity or revenue levels. The M. D. Anderson case study, presented later in this book, is a situation where direct connection was not possible and the effort ROI was based on differentials from historical levels.

Because this model does not connect the marketing effort directly to the actual usage, some organizations opt to put in a "safety valve" to account for market fluctuations and noise. For example, we might opt to count only volumes greater than 110% of the historical average for the past three years, assuming that anything from 100% to 110% was just a factor of normal market fluctuation.

Here are some generic examples of how to use historical baselines as the basis for determining the results from a marketing effort:

- The Mid-Plains Diagnostic Imaging Center tracks referral volumes by doctor for the four-county area it serves. Mid-Plains recently added a 0.5 full-time equivalent (FTE) sales staff person and gave that individual a goal of reaching out to 100 physicians who have not sent any volumes to the center in the past two years. Since there is no direct connection mechanism available, Mid-Plains can only look at the change in volumes after the implementation of the sales effort. Since the historical volume (two years) from the target doctors is zero, the organization will count any increases as coming from the specific sales/liaison effort.

- West Coast University (WCU) has one of the very few proton devices for the treatment of prostate and other types of cancer. Historically WCU has promoted this program using media coverage and print advertising in publications that reach the desired demographics nationally. This past year, WCU opted to target five specific metropolitan areas with both geographically and demographically targeted promotions. Because of the history of national marketing efforts and limita-

A Marketer's Guide to Measuring ROI

tions on internal tracking systems (e.g., the call center), the organization believes it will be challenging to connect inquiries and usage directly to the specific targeted efforts. It opts to look at actual inquiries and volumes in each of the five markets over the historical averages (for three prior years) coming from those markets. In one case the historical average was five cases per year from a certain market. In the 12 months after the targeted promotion, the organization saw 31 cases from that targeted market. The gain was considered to be 26 cases.

- Retirement State Medical Center (RSMC) develops a multimodality effort aimed at seniors in the area to drive interest in and utilization of orthopedic surgery for knee replacement, hip replacement, and related services. Because of the nature of the marketing effort and the lack of resources to have a single point of contact for tracking, RSMC opts to look at increases in volumes over the level seen in the 12 months prior to the initiation of the marketing effort. In order to allow for market fluctuation and outside influences, RSMC decides to accept all volumes over 105% of the level seen in the prior year as coming from the marketing work. In the prior year, RSMC performed 420 knee replacement surgeries. As a result, all volumes over 440 knee replacement surgeries would be counted as a result of marketing initiatives.

Another approach to tracking the impact of a marketing effort is the use of a control group. In this situation, one known group receives the impact of the marketing effort while another group (ideally equal in size and demographic mix) does not. Returns from the two groups are tracked using identification information such as name, address, gender, age, etc.

The use of a control group has some limitations, however, as it can only work where we can be assured that the group that did not get the marketing communications was indeed not impacted by the marketing effort. Modalities such as media placements, radio, print, television, and outdoor generally don't work well with a control-group approach. Efforts that do lend themselves to such an approach include direct mail, e-mail blasts, highly targeted community events, and sales/liaison contacts.

The following is an example of an effective use of a control group:

- Hospital S contracts with a vendor to develop and distribute a direct-mail effort aimed at getting consumers in a specific age/gender group to participate in an online cardiology health screening. The mailing is sent to 25,000 households where one member meets the desired demographic. Another 25,000 households are used as a control group. Over the course of 12 months the hospital tracks the number of individuals taking the test and eventually using heart-related services at Hospital S versus the level of usage out of the control group. The differential between the two groups is considered by executive management to come as a result of the impact of the marketing effort.

As part of the effort ROI measurement process, one of the key up-front assumptions is how the volumes coming from the marketing effort are going to be tracked. If the methodology is to look at levels over the historical volumes, a consensus needs to be established as to (a) what the historical level is and (b) whether there is going to be any kind of "safety valve" factor of, say, 5 or 10%.

Step 5: Determine how long to measure

The measurement we are talking about in this book is return on investment. The term investment implies a long period of time. One of the biggest challenges to successful healthcare effort ROI measurement is the failure to measure for a long enough period of time to allow for (a) impact on the key audiences, and (b) usage to be needed or for patients to get through the clinical system.

In the rush to meet fiscal-year objectives, provider organizations sometimes lack the patience and discipline to give the marketing effort a chance to work. Later in the book we will look at an example of an occupational health program that opted to cut off the measurement of effort ROI at the end of the calendar year, even though a significant part of the marketing work did not take place until that fall. As a result, the ROI was likely understated.

 As noted previously, each organization must decide what is "right" in terms of how long to measure. That said, I would recommend that no measurement be done for fewer than six months after the start of a marketing initiative. In fact, the more appropriate measurement period is one year.

Also, if the measurement period is longer than one year it is a good idea to do interim measurements, perhaps every six months. It is asking a lot to assume that senior management will have the patience to wait two or more years for results without some feel for the success or failure on an interim basis.

Step 6A: Determine factors for new business

Some organizations believe that marketing efforts should bring in new patients and new volumes, and while this is difficult to define and measure, it is not an unreasonable viewpoint. The challenge, however, is to define what is meant by "new" patients. Here is the spectrum of possible measures for new patients, from the most liberal to the very (perhaps overly) conservative:

- **Liberal.** It doesn't matter if the patient has been there before or not. The organization will count any volume that can be connected to the marketing effort.

- **Middle-of-the-road liberal.** To be counted, a patient cannot have used the organization in a certain number of years (usually 2–3) for that specific clinical area only.

- **Middle-of-the-road conservative.** To be counted, a patient cannot have used the organization in a certain number of years (up to five years but usually 2–3 years) for any type of service.

- **Conservative.** Only patients who have never used the organization for healthcare services before are counted.

Author's note

In working on effort ROI tracking, I have seen all models applied at various points in time, though the most common is the middle-of-the-road liberal. Whichever model your organization uses, the decision on the assumption must be made up front, before the marketing initiative is started and well before any attempts at measurement are made.

The liberal model is a good approach for a totally new program or new organization with no track record of historical patients. Meanwhile, the fully conservative approach has a lot of problems and really should not be considered. The first problem is determining if an individual has ever been a patient at the organization. Most organizations only keep records for so long, after all. More importantly, in many markets this approach excludes all but a very small percentage of the population, leaving very few candidates who might be considered as coming as a result of the marketing work.

Step 6B: Factors for 'business we would have gotten anyway'

Many healthcare marketing professionals have heard the refrain "we would have gotten that business anyway," implying that the work of marketing had nothing to do with driving usage of the provider. While some of that is organizational culture clash and politically related, there is some degree of truth in the statement. Just by existing and being open a provider will get some volumes. And if the specific program has been around for a while, it had a patient base prior to the initiation of any marketing work. So it is quite reasonable to apply a factor for "business we would have gotten anyway" to any effort ROI measurement. The trick is how to apply that factor. As with most of the other assumptions, there is no absolute right or wrong here. Here are some examples of models used by providers to factor out some degree of business that the organization might have received without the marketing effort:

- **No factor.** In this case, the organization decides to apply no factor for business they would have gotten anyway and accepts that all volumes coming in (in total or over historical levels) came as a result of the marketing effort. This approach is probably most appropriate when a program is new and thus there is no historical volume level. For example, Hospital A starts a deep-brain stimulation for the treatment of Parkinson's disease. For the first two years, all volumes coming in are assumed to come from the marketing efforts used and no factor for business they would have gotten anyway is applied.

- **Safety margin factor.** As discussed earlier, in many cases there is no system in place to connect a certain marketing activity directly to specific patient volume. In those instances, organizations often consider volumes over historical patterns to have come from the marketing effort (assuming no other extraneous factors such as the closure of a competitive service). However, to allow for market noise and a degree of business they would have gotten anyway, the organization decides to establish a factor of perhaps 5%–15% over the historical level before the marketing effort results kick in.

- **Existing market share.** Perhaps the simplest factor to use—and the one likely to cause the least debate—is to remove a percentage from new volumes equal to the most recent level of known market share. This approach is most viable when the program being marketed is long established and has a track record of volumes at the provider organization. So if Hospital B has a 25% market share in the service area for orthopedic surgery, all volumes attributed to a specific marketing effort might be reduced by 25% to allow for business they would have gotten anyway.

 A Marketer's Guide to Measuring ROI

The factors for new business and business we would have gotten anyway are clearly related but still independent factors. In order to develop an effort ROI measurement, the organization needs to decide whether it will apply both, one or the other, or neither. Again, there is no right approach. An organization that opts to count new patients as those who have not been there in three years might then not worry about a factor for business they would have gotten anyway. Or the organization might not bother trying to track whether the patient is new, instead taking all volume connected to the marketing effort and then subtracting a percentage equal to its current market share.

Lean toward being more conservative. If a marketing effort can show a respectable effort ROI by restricting itself to a reasonable definition of new patients and also factor out some likely business they would have gotten anyway, the credibility of the effort is significantly enhanced.

Step 7: The financial side—net revenues and cost of services provided

While steps 1–6 dealt with marketing costs, tracking, and key assumptions, the last step in the process is to determine two key financial factors—how much in the way of net revenues did we get from the marketing-driven volume and what was the cost of services provided?

Net revenues

Effort ROI is based on revenues collected from patient volumes deemed to have come as a result of the specific marketing effort net of contractual allowances and bad debts. *If the money is not collected by the organization, it does not count as part of effort ROI.* Using net revenues creates a number of possible challenges for marketing staff:

- **Gaining access to net revenue figures.** For a variety of reasons, net revenue by service or program is not readily available outside of the financial function. In other words, the information exists but is not openly shared. Fortunately, this is a situation that seems to be changing in most organizations.

- **Determining specific net revenues from specific patients or cases.** In ideal circumstances, we have the capability to connect a specific patient (and the revenues from that patient) to a specific marketing effort. If we succeed in capturing Mr. Jones with our marketing, and the resulting surgery gives us net revenues of $19,375, we can apply that figure to the ROI calculation. In less-than-ideal (but perhaps more common) circumstances, we can only measure that overall volume in a particular clinical area went up by, say, 12% in the year after we initiated the marketing effort. The problem is we don't know specifically which patients made up the 12%. So to be able to calculate an effort ROI, we will need to know an average net revenue for cases in this clinical area of service.

- **Time delay in getting net revenue figures.** It isn't unusual for payment for specific services to be delayed for two months or more after the service is received. Even then, it can take internal accounting systems a while to track and record the revenues. So it may be a while after the cut-off date for the tracking of effort ROI before the calculations can be completed.

- **The revenue stream can continue for quite a while.** For some services (such as a knee replacement) the revenue stream from care is fairly

A Marketer's Guide to Measuring ROI

finite and short term. For other services (such as diabetes or cancer) the treatment process can go on for quite a while, and so can the revenue stream. At some point there is a need to cut off the information flow (e.g., level of net revenues) in order to calculate effort ROI. In turn, however, leadership needs to recognize that the ROI result may be a bit understated because more returns may come in after the measurement point.

 The statement above is not meant to imply that there isn't an important place for charity care among healthcare providers. Charity care is a crucial part of our culture and should be encouraged. But effort ROI is a business model meant to measure the financial return from a specific marketing or business development activity. As a result, it should be used only with actual collected revenues.

Gross charges should not be used to calculate effort ROI—period. In my work on ROI tracking over the past decade I have encountered a fair number of instances where the measurement of the impact of marketing was made using gross charges. The reason this financial figure was used is fairly simple—it was the easiest figure to get. But gross charges can significantly overstate effort ROI because we often take 20%, 30%, or more off for contractual allowances and bad debt. Since it is widely known in the healthcare field that gross charges are a relatively meaningless figure, any ROI result based on gross charges is not likely to have much credibility.

Cost of services sold

The final key element in the development of an effort ROI is the application of a factor for the cost of services sold. This is an essential step in the calculation of a complete, detailed effort ROI analysis. Without factoring for cost of services sold the ROI is overstated, as no organization collects and keeps every dollar it bills—a very large portion goes out for expenses.

While every organization treats its accounting a bit differently, expenses generally fall into three categories: direct variable, indirect variable, and fixed. Each of these expense categories can be defined (in very general terms) as follows:

- **Direct variable expenses.** Expenses that vary with volume and are directly connected to patient utilization of services (e.g., clinical staff time, food, drugs, surgical supplies, linens, etc.)

- **Indirect variable expenses.** Expenses that vary to a degree with patient utilization or are at least allocated via some patient usage formula (e.g., nonclinical staff time, non-clinical supplies, etc.)

- **Fixed (overhead) expenses.** Expenses that essentially stay the same whether there are any patients or not (e.g., bond payments, depreciation, utilities, malpractice insurance, payments in lieu of taxes, etc.)

The effort ROI calculation must include direct variable expenses (deducted from net revenues) in order to be a rigorous assessment of the return on a marketing investment. Some organizations may also opt to include indirect variable expenses (see the M. D. Anderson case study later in the book).

The factor for direct expenses should be measurable as a percentage of net

A Marketer's Guide to Measuring ROI

revenues and should be available from the organization's financial function. In some cases this figure may be a "best-guess" estimate, but even if it is, it should be used in the calculation. In addition, it is highly likely that the direct variable expense percentage will vary by clinical service or program. In other words, it will be different for obstetrics, cardiology, or outpatient diagnostic imaging.

 Unless the marketing effort is so successful that the organization has to build a new facility or acquire capital equipment to handle the volume, fixed or overhead expenses should not be included in effort ROI calculation. Given the profit margins of most healthcare provider organizations, including overhead usually leaves no more than 10% (and usually much less) of net revenues after expenses. At that rate, no marketing effort will ever show a positive ROI. If a marketing effort works and brings in new patient volumes and new revenues, those revenues (net of direct costs) should be considered contribution margin to the overhead costs of the organization.

How is ROI from a marketing effort actually calculated?

How is ROI from a marketing effort actually calculated?

The effort ROI formula

The actual formula for measuring effort-driven return on investment (ROI) is fairly straightforward. You start with net revenue (i.e., revenues collected after contractual obligations and bad debt), subtract cost of services sold, and divide by all appropriate marketing cost elements, including allocated staff time. As a mathematical formula, it looks like this:

$$\text{ROI\%} = \frac{\text{Net revenue} - \text{marketing expense}}{\text{Marketing expense}} \times 100$$

An example of effort ROI

Let's illustrate this formula with a simple example.

Organizational background

River City Occupational Health Services (RCOHS) is a joint venture between Memorial Medical Center and a group of independent occupational health physicians. The organization has four provider sites and is generally considered to be the leading occupational health provider in the River City area.

Marketing effort

The current marketing portfolio for RCOHS includes paid advertising in the local business weekly, a Web site, a sales force of three people (who routinely make both cold calls and qualified-lead contacts), and periodic "business breakfast" educational programs, supported by direct-mail invitations and e-mails to an internally developed list of contacts.

Twice a year there is a local industrial trade show held at the River City Convention Center. This event, sponsored by the local chamber of commerce, allows local businesses to show off their capabilities for other businesses—especially in the heavier industrial/service trades.

Historically, RCOHS has not participated in these trade shows, but decided to try this strategy for one year (two shows) to see how effective it might be. Participation in these single-day trade shows involves creating a display booth, buying giveaway materials, paying a participation fee, and sales staff time to man the booth.

ROI analysis information and assumptions

Marketing effort elements:
- Trade show booth
- Trade show giveaway materials

- Entrance fees
- Staff time
- **Total cost = $11,500**

Time period for tracking results:

- Only through the end of the calendar year in question. (Note: The trade shows were held in the spring and fall of each year. As a result, cutting off the tracking by December 31 likely limited the measurement of the return from the fall effort.)

Tracking methodology:

- Any time a firm signs a "letter of service" with RCOHS, the source of the new business is recorded. In turn, an internal database tracks all patient volumes by the source of request for service. Patients at RCOHS can't just walk in off the street. They have to have a referral approved by the payer—which is the firm they work for. Thus RCOHS can tell with certainty (and fairly quickly) the source of all patient volumes.

Factor for new patients to the organization:

- In this case, a factor for new patients is not relevant except to note that before any company inquired at the fair and then signed a letter of service, RCOHS would not have gotten any occupational health business from them.

Factor for business would have gotten anyway:

- In this case, the situation is the same as for determining new patients. These firms did not send cases to RCOHS prior to the industrial fair and the subsequent sales call and letter of service, and so there really is no factor for "business we would have gotten anyway."

Results/revenues/costs of services provided:
- Number of inquiries coming from the industrial fairs: 14
- Number converting to clients in the calendar year: 6
- Services revenues generated by December 31: $41,500
- Cost of services sold factor: 40%
- Net revenues from volumes generated from the industrial fair: $24,900

Effort ROI calculation

$$\text{ROI\%} = \frac{\text{Net revenue} - \text{marketing expense}}{\text{Marketing expense}} \times 100$$

$$\text{ROI\%} = \frac{(\$24,900 - \$11,500)}{\$11,500} \times 100$$

$$\text{ROI percent} = 116\%$$

The leadership of RCOHS opted to set the time frame as the fiscal year (in this case the calendar year). As a result, the measurement of ROI was cut off for the second of the two industrial fairs only 90 or so days after the fair was over. This was probably not enough time to really see the impact of the marketing effort. In all likelihood, if RCOHS had extended the analysis for another 90–180 days, the effort ROI would have improved noticeably.

This brings up an important point: You must not only determine what time period you will use to track results, but you must also make sure that this time frame is realistic and will give you an accurate picture of the financial impact of your marketing effort. This is especially important in a healthcare setting, when patients don't always get to decide when they need your services.

A note on the formula for ROI

There are two schools of thought on the formula for ROI. One uses the multiplication factor of 100 and the other does not. In the former case, an ROI of 100% essentially is breakeven—the marketing effort generated just enough new revenue to cover the cost of the marketing effort. In the latter case, an ROI of 0 is breakeven. Neither is necessarily right or wrong, but the key is to be consistent. It could get very confusing to mix the methodologies and end up with one effort that has an ROI of 109% and other with an ROI of 45%—and, in reality, the 45% return is better because the multiplication factor was not used.

Another example of effort ROI

While discussion and formulas can be helpful, I find that examples are the best way to demonstrate the usage of effort ROI in a provider setting. So let's look at one more example. In this case the marketing effort does not involve any expenditures specifically for advertising or communications purposes.

Organizational background

Mountain Valley General Hospital (MVGH) owns a diagnostic imaging (DI) center in a nearby physician's office building (which it also owns). This center offers a range of services, including x-rays, mammography, ultrasound, CT scan, MRI, etc. Historically the facility has been open 8:30 a.m. to 6:00 p.m., Monday through Friday, and 9:00 a.m. to 1:00 p.m. on Saturdays.

The DI center's competition is a physician-owned facility about five miles away, and a joint venture facility run by another hospital about eight miles away. In addition, outpatient services are available at the two local hospitals, though neither can offer the convenience of the freestanding sites. Anecdotally, the managers at the DI center have gotten increasing feedback from their clients that coming during the day is inconvenient, and having an after-work option to get prescribed tests would be a significant attraction.

Marketing effort

The center decides to expand its hours of operation to 8:00 p.m. on Mondays, Tuesdays, Wednesdays, and Thursdays. This expansion is promoted through existing channels to key audiences (area physicians, local consumers, etc.). The key concern of the managers of the DI center is whether this effort

A Marketer's Guide to Measuring ROI

would net new volumes or whether it would just cannibalize existing volumes by giving the current patients more convenient times to come for service.

ROI analysis information and assumptions

Marketing effort elements:

- Expansion of hours

- Promotion through existing channels (newsletters, Website, e-mail, and word of mouth via physician liaisons)

- Total cost = $24,000 (additional labor and estimated power costs)

Time period for tracking results:

- Results were tracked for six months after the initiation of the extended hours of operation

- Note: ROI could not be calculated for 10 months (four months after the cutoff point) due to limitations in the ability to get revenue figures

Tracking methodology:

- Tracking efforts focused on looking at total volumes and revenues coming to the DI center in the period prior to the change in hours and the period after

- In addition, management looked carefully at whether there was any significant decline in volumes during the original operating hours (8:30 a.m. to 6:00 p.m.)

Factors for new patients and business they would have gotten anyway:

- Management felt that the effort required to determine if the additional volumes were new patients was not an important issue, though some informal efforts would be made to see if volumes came from any new referral sources

- Management also felt that there was no practical way to consider business they would have gotten anyway

- Overall, the analysis would look at whether the total volumes and revenues grew and whether there was a decline during the original operating hours, which would signify a shift in usage, not a gain

Results/revenues/costs of services provided:

- At the end of the six months, management determined that revenues increased by an average of about $1,500 per day (actual collections)

- There were only minor declines in volumes during the original operating hours, and these were more than made up by the gains during the extended hours

- Informally, they determined that some referrals (perhaps one or two a day) were now coming from physicians outside of the medical office building who had not sent cases there in the past. Brief registration surveys done with patients showed that the driving reason was the convenience of being able to come after hours

- Revenues generated in six months: $150,000

- Cost of services sold factor: 55%

- Net revenues: $67,500

Effort ROI calculation:

$$ROI\% = \frac{\text{Net revenue} - \text{Marketing expense}}{\text{Marketing expense}} \times 100$$

$$ROI\% = \frac{(\$67,500 - \$24,000)}{\$24,000} \times 100$$

$$ROI \text{ percent} = 181\%$$

Is there only one way to report ROI?

5

Is there only one way to report ROI?

Three ways to report ROI

There are actually three ways to report return on investment (ROI). The diagnostic imaging example from the previous chapter is the most common approach, which is the percentage methodology. Other options include a ratio approach and a time to break even approach.

To illustrate the ROI reporting methodologies, let's use some simple results information from a hypothetical hospital marketing effort:

- Net revenues (after direct costs) from volumes coming from the marketing effort = $50,000

- Cost of the marketing effort = $20,000

Model 1: Effort ROI in a percentage format

$$\text{ROI\%} = \frac{\text{Net revenue} - \text{Marketing expense}}{\text{Marketing expense}} \times 100$$

$$\text{ROI\%} = \frac{(\$50{,}000 - \$20{,}000)}{\$20{,}000} \times 100$$

$$\text{ROI percent} = 150\%$$

The percentage approach is the method that is most commonly used and referred to in management literature—therefore it is most easily recognized. I recommend that you use it for any provider-based effort ROI analysis.

$$ROI = \text{Net return} \div \text{marketing expense}$$

$$ROI = \$50{,}000 \div \$20{,}000$$

$$ROI = 2.5 \text{ to } 1$$

Model 2: Effort ROI in a ratio format

This format for reporting effort ROI is merely a statistical restating of the information derived from the first model. It is a viable way of reporting ROI, but the first model is still preferred.

Model 3: Effort ROI in a time to break even format

$$ROI = (\text{Marketing expense} \div \text{net return}) \times 12 \text{ months}$$

$$ROI = (\$20{,}000 \div \$50{,}000) \times 12 \text{ months}$$

$$ROI = 4.8 \text{ months}$$

 This is perhaps the most esoteric of the three reporting models. It makes for an interesting variation if you want to track how long it takes (weeks, months, etc.) to get a return on a marketing investment. Since this is very rarely used and really focuses more on the time period than the level of return, this approach probably has very limited utility in a provider setting.

Why is it so important that we take a rigorous approach to effort ROI?

Why is it so important that we take a rigorous approach to effort ROI?

A question of credibility

Marketing efforts have many positive impacts. An internal marketing campaign might boost employee morale. A branding campaign might cause an upswing in preference share. The cardiology department might get a bump in volume after a television ad for the cardiology service line campaign runs on local cable stations. But to call these results a return on investment (ROI) undermines the credibility of true effort ROI and, in turn, the credibility of the provider marketing function.

Effort ROI (by the nature of the definition provided in Chapter 1) implies that we can measure the net revenue derived from business (patient volumes) that can be connected to a specific marketing effort. If there are no measurable revenues, there is no ROI. If we can't factor out a reasonable degree of business we would have gotten anyway, we have, at best, an overstated ROI. If we use gross charges instead of net revenues, we definitely have an overstated ROI. And if we can't factor out costs of services sold, we have an incomplete

ROI (though it can be argued that we are at least headed down the appropriate path).

Let's go back to the Introduction of this book and look again at Case A. The hospital hired an external public relations firm at a cost of $65,000 to secure media coverage for them. The firm was quite successful and provided a report to the client that showed that they had obtained coverage that, had they purchased the same number of column inches or radio minutes, would have cost $142,000. Their report called this result a return on investment for the public relations effort. In truth, this really was an excellent return in terms of value received for the money spent. But because there were no revenues generated by the media coverage gained, there was no effort ROI as we have discussed it in this book.

Unfortunately for the marketing function, the leadership of the hospital (lead by the financial function) recognized that there was no real ROI from this media relations effort. As a result, the value of the effort was minimized and credibility was lost. The effort should have been portrayed as what it was—a success in terms of (a) getting specific levels of media coverage and (b) a good "buy" in terms of the amount of media coverage in excess of the pure dollars spent. But it should not have been portrayed as ROI.

At this point some of my readers may be rolling their eyes a bit and wondering if I am being way too picky about this. Perhaps I am, but I have a good reason to be. Healthcare marketing professionals have worked hard over the past 30 years to create a viable management position within the provider sector. A good part of that effort has focused on coming up with ways to show the value of marketing to the organization. The very fact that we are now discussing rigorous measurements of trackable, hard effort ROI says a great deal about the progress of our profession. Any use of the effort ROI measure in a way that doesn't follow the parameters outlined in earlier chapters undermines this progress.

I would ask the reader to understand that the intent of the last statement is not to suggest that any ROI-related activity that doesn't go to the full extreme is not worth the bother. Just the opposite is true. Partial ROI efforts go a long way toward showing that (a) marketing as a function is concerned about measurement and (b) that there is a viable return for marketing resources. In addition, work that goes part of the way to a full effort ROI analysis gains the organization experience that will come in handy when the impediment to full ROI measurement (perhaps the availability of direct-cost percentages) is removed.

Are there other metrics we should consider when we measure our marketing efforts?

Are there other metrics we should consider when we measure our marketing efforts?

Alternatives to effort ROI

I am a strong proponent of the use of hard metrics for any level of provider marketing plans—from medical groups to service lines to single hospitals to multiunit systems. Effort return on investment (ROI) is a desirable measure to add to provider marketing plans, but, as we have discussed, it isn't easy to do. And, truth be told, most providers will not be able to use effort ROI for a majority of their specific marketing efforts.

There are generally two categories of metrics outside of effort ROI. The first category is operational or production-oriented metrics. The second category is result- or outcomes-oriented metrics. Following are some examples of each category.

Operational/production metrics
- **Did the annual report get out on time?** Due to the attention the annual report often gets from the senior leadership, getting it out on time on a

regular basis can be an impressive indication of operational efficiency (or the fact that your marketing staff did without a lot of sleep).

• **How many collateral pieces were produced?** This measurement should be used with a degree of caution since it begs the question as to whether the collaterals were needed. But it is at the very least a measure of how busy the marketing/public relations function was during the past year.

• **How many media placements were actually picked up and used by local media outlets?** Noting how many media stories were sent out is one measure, but the more effective one is how many were actually placed and how much coverage they actually generated.

• **How many listeners do we have for our weekly health-issues cable television talk show?** This can be challenging to measure since cable outlets often have limited viewer information. One methodology is to include some questions on this issue in the annual service-area consumer survey.

• **How many speakers bureau requests did we have?** Speakers bureaus are relatively low cost, but a highly effective (if not very cutting edge) marketing technique for providers. Track how many inquiries came in, how many events your speakers actually participated in, and (ideally) how many people actually attended these events.

• **What is the advertising recall level for our advertising versus our competitors?** Advertising recall is not an effort ROI measurement but it is a

A Marketer's Guide to Measuring ROI

useful tool to track the degree to which your advertising is gaining and holding public attention. This can be measured via periodic service-area consumer surveys.

- **How many participants did we have at our community events such as health screenings?** The level of community event efforts by hospitals, medical groups, and other providers varies widely. If this strategy is used, however, a minimal level of tracking that should be implemented is to record how many people actually participated.

- **How many calls did we get to the call center?** Call center software has been part of our industry since the early 1980s, and by its very nature it allows for significant levels of tracking (and can be a great help in the tracking component of effort ROI). While the total number of calls is a very basic measurement, moving to the next level would involve tracking what the calls were for (physician referral, program registration, order fulfillment, prescription refills, after-hours physician office coverage, etc.).

- **How much activity did our Web site receive?** As with call centers, the Web site software contains myriad ways to track usage. Very basic measurements include the number of Web hits, the pages viewed, the time spent on each page, the number of unique users, etc. Perhaps more important for marketing purposes is measuring the degree of interactivity (the number of class registrations, the sales on the company store portion of the site, the number of job applications, etc.).

- **What is the size of our e-mail database?** At this writing, provider organizations are just now starting to recognize the power of being able to send targeted promotional information via e-mail. While this approach lends itself to effort ROI tracking, a very basic production measurement is the overall size of the e-mail database. These databases cannot be bought (at this time) but have to be developed by soliciting voluntary submission of e-mail addresses via Web inquiries, sign-ups for classes and events, registration for services, etc.

Results/outcomes goals

- **Volumes (admissions, days, visits, etc.).** Probably the most basic outcomes measure in the field but still a critical one.

- **Market share.** Most organizations consider this to be a key measure of marketing success. That said, moving market share should not automatically be associated with successful ROI. It is quite possible to increase share without generating positive revenues, depending upon the service in question and the payer mix of the new patient volumes.

- **Changes in payer mix.** As noted in the market share section, gaining share or volume may not be enough due to the nature of our complicated payment and reimbursement system. As a result, it is important to track movements in payer mix by service.

- **Top-of-mind awareness.** Which hospital comes to mind first among key audiences? This is a basic but key measurement of the brand strength of your organization, measured via a periodic survey of service-area consumers (or other key audience if appropriate).

 A Marketer's Guide to Measuring ROI

- **Overall and clinical service preference.** Which hospital is preferred by area consumers overall, which ones do they prefer for specific services, and which ones would they not prefer to use? Overall and clinical service performance is measured via a periodic service-area consumer survey.

- **Organizational image.** This is a key non-ROI metric. What do key audiences (consumers, civic leaders, referral sources, our own employees, etc., think about us?) Organizational image can be measured via the use of quantitative research such as service-area consumer surveys. At the consumer level, possible measurements include perceived quality, overall best in the market, whether a consumer would refer this hospital to others, etc.

- **Number of contracts closed.** For some programs (e.g., occupational health) a key measurement is whether we closed the contract with a purchaser.

- **Number of referrals generated and/or number of active referral sources.** This is a crucial category of metrics, especially for more highly specialized providers such as tertiary medical groups (cardiology, neurosurgery, etc.) and teaching/university medical centers. It can be a challenging metric to achieve, and as a result it is not universally found in our field.

- **Number of memberships.** A fairly simple measure, but a key one if you have a program that involves actual membership, such as a fitness center.

- **Key audience satisfaction with services.** This is another key metric that perhaps is not directly related to effort ROI but certainly can have an impact on the potential for ROI. Key audience satisfaction is measured statistically via user surveys and qualitatively via interviews, focus groups, and observational research.

- **Number of lives captured (capitated arrangements).** Capitation as a payment model has faded since its heyday in the 1990s but it hasn't gone away. If a component of your organization still relies upon capitated lives (such as an IPA or an employed primary care group) then tracking the number of lives captured or retained is a viable measure. It is also one that can be readily expanded into an effort ROI analysis.

     A Marketer's Guide to Measuring ROI

If I can show a really good effort ROI, can I get an increase in the marketing budget?

If I can show a really good effort ROI, can I get an increase in the marketing budget?

Your marketing department has developed an award-winning direct-mail campaign aimed at driving target markets to participate in an online cardiology screening. A noticeable number of participants end up getting referrals to your cardiologists and eventually end up using heart-related care at your hospital. You can directly connect the users because of unique identifier numbers, you can measure business you would have expected anyway, etc. The quintessential effort ROI tracking situation.

After 12 months of tracking you can show a 425% return on an expenditure of $300,000. Great job! Isn't this justification for increasing the marketing budget? After all, if we got a 425% return on spending $300,000, imagine what we could do with $1 million.

If you do have this kind of success and want to pursue a larger marketing budget, I'll be happy to back you up. But truth be told, it isn't quite that easy or simple. All markets are finite in size and the return on marketing efforts is not a never-ending straight line going up and to the right. Eventually the curve starts getting steeper and steeper as you gain more and more of the market. At some point you will saturate the potential for heart screenings and follow-up heart care in your market, and the effort ROI will drop significantly, if not turn negative.

How to tell when the end is near

Since effort ROI in the healthcare provider setting is so new, there really are no models to use to know what is a poor, average, or exceptional effort ROI—and there are no models to tell you when you've about tapped out what you can get. In lieu of that let me suggest some possible warning signs:

- You tracked a specific effort for 12 months and the overall ROI was good, but the significant majority of the new volume came in the first four months, and the level of inquiries and volumes has declined steadily since then.

- You plan to track the effort ROI for two years, with incremental measurements every six months. The level of effort ROI steadily drops each six-month period, though it remains positive throughout.

    A Marketer's Guide to Measuring ROI

Is ROI measurement a useful tool only if you gain volumes?

Is ROI measurement a useful tool only if you gain volumes?

There are times when there really is no room to gain new volumes, or we use marketing just to hold onto the volumes and share we have. The question about what to do in that situation first came up during one of my presentations on this topic. The question and the subsequent discussion led to the concept of what I will call "reverse" effort return on investment (ROI); in other words, tracking the ROI from marketing efforts that successfully allow an organization to hold on to volumes or share in the face of severe competition or adverse circumstances. Some examples of severe competition or adverse circumstances might include:

- In a two-hospital market, Hospital A recruits away a key three-physician OB practice from Hospital B (and this includes hiring the OB physicians into the employed physician group owned by Hospital A). This group accounts for 20% of the OB volume at Hospital B.

- A nurse is discovered conducting "mercy" killings of elderly patients in Hospital C's intensive care unit. This story is page one in the local newspaper and at the top of the news on all three of the local television stations.

- Dr. Jones is a nationally known orthopedic surgeon and is the lead physician in a key five-physician orthopedic group. He practices almost exclusively at Hospital D. Unfortunately, during a skiing trip he has an accident. He will recover from his injuries but it will be six months before he can get back into the surgical schedule—and his group members are at capacity and can't cover 100% of his cases.

In each of these cases the hospital in question faces some very real and potentially very serious volume losses. In each case, the hospital scrambles to do damage control through the investment of communications and non-communications marketing resources (including physician recruitment). In all three cases, the hospitals were able to minimize the losses to a level much less than what was initially projected. So can they measure a reverse ROI on these efforts—a return on preventing what's very likely to be a loss? I believe they can, in almost the same manner as was described in previous chapters for normal effort ROI.

The primary change is in the up-front assumptions and measurements. Instead of tracking the volumes coming from a specific marketing effort and/or the level of increase over a historical average, the organization now must come up with a consensus assumption on how much volume they expect to lose—and then measure how much of that loss is avoided through the marketing effort.

A Marketer's Guide to Measuring ROI

An example of volume retention ROI

Let's illustrate this using the first case, where Hospital A recruits away the OB group from Hospital B. The initial projection shows that Hospital B will lose 500 deliveries per year from this defection, phased in over time as the OB group disengages and moves over to Hospital A. Within 48 hours of the notification of the move, Hospital B puts a recovery plan into place. Elements within this plan include:

- Recruiting an additional OB physician into a two-doctor OB/GYN group employed by the hospital

- Immediately making minor cosmetic improvements to the physical area of the OB postpartum unit, originally scheduled for six months later

- Offering free meal trays to fathers visiting new mothers and babies

- Introducing a series of public education seminars for first-time mothers, with tips on handling new infants, and other OB/newborn-related topics

- Sending targeted mailings to all patients who had used the defecting physicians for OB services at Hospital B in the past three years, encouraging them to use Hospital B again if they have another child (but not directly encouraging them to change doctors)

- Designing and implementing an OB advertising campaign (print, radio, billboard)

Over the course of the next 18 months, the organization tracks the level of births against what it anticipated losing from the loss of the key OB group. Instead of losing 20% of its OB volume, the organization loses only 8% during the measurement period. That's a loss prevented of 280 OB cases.

In this instance the effort ROI measurement process would be the same as described in Chapter 4, but the net revenues would be figured from the volume that was prevented from leaving the organization. While this must be recognized as not being new revenues, the fact that the marketing efforts prevented a significant loss is very valuable and can be measured as part of an effort ROI analysis.

A Marketer's Guide to Measuring ROI

So where do we start?

So where do we start?

I'm often asked what the right "level" of effort return on investment (ROI) tracking is for the marketing function of a hospital or health system or medical group. Should we be doing ROI tracking on half of our efforts? A quarter? Ten percent? Since measuring ROI is relatively new to healthcare, there are no industry standards at this time. It may be a number of years before we have enough usage of effort ROI tracking to be able to establish a standard.

That said, I recommend to all provider-based marketing functions that they start small and gain experience. Build one hard, rigorous, effort ROI measurement process into the current fiscal year's marketing plan. Then add two or three more the next year. Build up the usage to the point where you can show solid effort ROI measurements on the majority of larger (higher resource usage) tactics designed to drive volumes. But be aware that this could take a few years to accomplish—and perhaps the dedication of part of a full-time equivalent (FTE) to manage the overall tracking process. This implementation cost must be taken into account as there is no value in spending your effort ROI (in staff time and tracking systems) to measure your effort ROI.

There is no perfect place to begin, as the market and program mix will vary for every provider organization. Some common elements in programs that I would recommend considering for marketing departments just starting out include the following:

- Services that are either elective and/or have a high degree of consumer participation in the decision to use them.

- Marketing efforts involving a single modality (such as only direct mail or only a radio campaign). This can be modified if the organization is willing to examine the ROI on the overall marketing effort and not worry about trying to get returns on different marketing elements.

- A service and a marketing effort where there is already a solid tracking methodology in place and/or it will be fairly simple to create such a methodology.

- A service where the financial arm can provide relatively timely feedback on volumes and revenues collected, and where they can reasonably provide a figure for direct-cost percentages.

A good place to begin

Examples of specific campaigns that lend themselves well to an initial foray into measuring effort ROI based on the guidelines in previous chapters include:

A Marketer's Guide to Measuring ROI

- **Elective eye (LASIK) or plastic surgery procedures.** University Hospital A (with an employed ophthalmology faculty group) promotes new LASIK eye-care capabilities and a "price special" both on its Web site and via an e-mail blast.

- **Screening efforts for cancer** (e.g., colon-rectal cancer screening kits distributed via local public outlets). Hospital B distributes colon-rectal cancer testing kits via its own regional outpatient sites and a local chain of pharmacies.

- **Occupational health services.** An independent occupational health program starts advertising regularly in the local business weekly via the creation of a workplace health tip column.

- **Hip- and knee-replacement surgery.** In a joint venture, a large orthopedic surgery group and Hospital C start a series of hip- and knee-replacement educational programs at breakfast meetings held at upscale developments for people age 55 and older.

- **Specialized mental health/dependency services.** A nationally recognized mental health program starts a residential treatment service for impaired professionals (doctors, lawyers, Fortune 1000 executives, etc.). In one marketing effort, a three-part direct-mail effort is implemented, aimed at senior HR executives in larger firms across the country.

- **Fitness club membership.** Hospital D owns two fitness centers in a joint venture with a national firm. Hospital D also has a 30,000 member senior club for individuals age 60 and older. The hospital develops a special pricing package for non-peak hours and promotes that package through mailings to senior-club members and in the senior-club newsletter.

- **Bariatric surgery.** A radio and print campaign promotes educational classes for bariatric surgery.

- **Emergency services.** Hospital E begins a concerted effort aimed at service-area emergency squads, attempting to repair historical ill will and educate squad members about the clinical capabilities at the hospital.

- **Capitated lives.** Apple Valley IPA, in cooperation with Hospital F, starts a health fair program for area businesses. This program is designed to be used during open enrollment periods when employees select their source of physician care for the following year.

- **Referral-source relations.** This is an exception to the guidelines noted previously, but it works as a starter for ROI tracking because the effort can be isolated to see if it worked. Hospital G has never had a formal physician-relations program. It starts by hiring one representative and targeting that representative at primary care physicians in its secondary/tertiary markets.

A Marketer's Guide to Measuring ROI

Is anything less than effort ROI worth doing?

Is anything less than effort ROI worth doing?

Any attempt at return on investment (ROI) measurement is worth doing, as long as the result doesn't create a seriously unrealistic picture of the impact of marketing. A tracking effort that can't quite be completed because cost of services sold information is not available is certainly heading down the right path. On the other hand, a measurement that uses gross charges instead of net revenue or that counts all of the volume coming into a program instead of the incremental gain over historical levels is likely detrimental in the long run, because it will damage credibility instead of enhancing it.

Examples of 'almost' ROI

Following are some examples of ROI tracking efforts that are on the right path, but not quite fully there yet.

The almost ROI of a consumer education effort

Southern Hospital conducts (with paid promotional support) a series of educational programs aimed at generating consumer interest in specific services and eventual usage of those services when appropriate. The seminars are a joint venture with specialists on the medical staff of the hospital. Southern has detailed information on marketing costs, and can track the net revenue (gross charges less contractual obligations) coming from patients who attended the seminars.

The organization has decided not to apply a factor for business it would have gotten anyway because of the nature of the clinical services involved. However, due to IT issues, the hospital cannot determine if these patients were new and cannot determine a reasonable factor for costs of services sold. So the effort ROI measurement is limited to net revenues coming from patients connected to the marketing effort, and direct-marketing costs.

This will result in an ROI measurement that is overstated, but the organization's leadership recognizes this and is willing to accept this partial ROI as a good first step in measurement efforts.

The almost ROI of a physician relations effort

Midwestern University Medical Center develops a multimodality marketing effort aimed at referring and potential referring physicians in a six-state region. The objective is to improve familiarity with a number of key quaternary programs and thus generate more direct referrals. The medical center can track the costs of the marketing effort (including support costs, such as additional physician-to-physician call center staff), the number of referrals coming in, and the net revenues generated.

At this time, however, the medical center has not applied a factor for business it would have gotten anyway nor for the direct cost of services sold. The

 A Marketer's Guide to Measuring ROI

former likely could be handled via an analysis of the number of cases historically coming from beyond the immediate metro area for the medical center, in lieu of having a viable referral source database. Information on direct costs needs to come from the organization's financial systems, and due to a change in systems, that can't be done for 6–12 months.

As in the previous example, however, the organization's leadership recognizes the problem and accepts the initial effort ROI as some indication of a gross contribution coming from the marketing effort.

The almost ROI of a physician referral line

Mid-South Health System has a centralized call center that supports physician referral program efforts for a number of hospitals in the system. The software from the call center program can be used to reconcile inquiries for physician referral to hospital utilization for inpatient and outpatient care. This reconciliation is conducted four times a year. The system has information on marketing costs, including the cost of promoting the referral service. In addition, the system applies a factor for business it would have gotten anyway via the use of market share by primary/secondary service areas for each hospital in the organization.

When effort ROI is calculated for the program, however, the financial division insists upon applying all costs—including fixed overhead. As a result, the cost of services sold factor is 92% of every net revenue dollar generated. In this situation, the effort ROI comes out negative, though not by a large amount.

This creates a challenge for the marketing function because it appears that the call center referral program loses money when in fact it would have a noticeably positive effort ROI if the cost of services sold were limited to the direct and even indirect variable costs of patients actually coming from the program. This is an example of well-done effort ROI undermined by unreasonable assumptions.

A Marketer's Guide to Measuring ROI

Case studies
in effort ROI

Case studies in effort ROI

Introduction to the case studies

In closing this book, I want to provide the reader with some recent examples of marketing-related effort return on investment (ROI) tracking. As you read these cases you will likely note that none of the ROI processes was done in exactly the same way. Each organization used somewhat different tracking mechanisms and assumptions related to new patients; business they would have gotten anyway; application of direct, indirect, and overhead costs; etc. Despite the differences in approach, all were able to track ROI from a marketing activity with a solid degree of rigor. In the spirit of truth in advertising, I was involved only with the M. D. Anderson effort.

There are five case studies in this section. They will look at the ROI on the following efforts:

1. A blog to educate consumers about bariatric surgery at Genesis Health System in Davenport, IA

2. A membership/benefit program aimed at women and heart disease for Covenant Medical Center in Saginaw, MI

3. A marketing effort to support a consumer education seminar on surgical and nonsurgical options for osteoarthritis hip and knee issues at the Cleveland Clinic Foundation in Cleveland

4. Another Cleveland Clinic effort: a newsletter targeted at pediatric referral sources—family physicians, general pediatricians, and specialty pediatricians

5. An extended advertising effort for M. D. Anderson Cancer Center in Houston that targeted two distinct metropolitan areas in Texas

Case study 1: Genesis Health System

Sources
Teresa Fraker, manager, bariatric surgery program at Genesis; Joyce Engelmann, manager of corporate communications and marketing for Genesis; and Ben Dillon, vice president of Geonetric.

Organizational background
Genesis Health System is a three-hospital system based in Davenport, IA. The organization provides healthcare services for consumers in the Quad Cities region (Davenport, Bettendorf, Moline, and Rock Island) and surrounding counties in Eastern Iowa and Western Illinois. Genesis is the leading provider in the region, with an overall inpatient market share of approximately 62%.

A Marketer's Guide to Measuring ROI

Primary competition for Genesis comes from the Trinity Health System, which also has three hospitals in the Quad Cities area.

Trinity Health System started the first bariatric surgery program in the Quad Cities area. Genesis Health System launched its program in September 2003.

Marketing effort

In March 2004, Genesis developed a bariatric surgery blog (with the help of its Web site consultant, Geonetric). It featured an actual Genesis bariatric surgery patient, who also happened to be an RN. She provided regular updates on her experiences before and after surgery, contributing to the blog for about a year before retiring for personal reasons. The Genesis staff recruited other bariatric surgery patients to create their own blogs and continue the public service and marketing effort. As of April 2007, the organization had two active bloggers, one a registered nurse and the other an amateur writer. Genesis did not pay any of the bloggers for their contributions.

The bariatric surgery blog is hosted on the Genesis Web site. Interested parties must register for the blog online by entering their name, e-mail address, ZIP code, age, and gender. This allows them to read the posts online or opt to receive an automatic e-mail detailing the new posts.

At the start of the effort, Genesis ran some paid advertising to promote the blog to interested consumers (see the section on marketing costs, later). This dedicated advertising effort was not repeated, but the blog is promoted through existing Genesis marketing channels.

Other marketing efforts used by Genesis to promote the bariatric surgery program include public relations/news coverage efforts, articles in *Genesis Today*, a community newsletter published by the organization, consumer educational classes; and a consumer Webcast.

Some relevant program statistics (as of April of 2007):

- Bariatric surgeries performed since the start of the blog: 347

- Consumers registered to read the blog or receive e-mail updates: 762

- Bariatric surgery patients who said the blog influenced their decision: 80

ROI analysis information and assumptions

Marketing effort elements:
- Blog development and maintenance

- Initial paid media promotion for the blog

Marketing costs:
- Blog development: $1,000

- Estimated staff time: $2,500

- Media advertising: $16,000

- Total: $19,500

A Marketer's Guide to Measuring ROI

Time period for tracking results:

- Tracking of results has been performed since the launch of the blog in March 2004 (about three years of data).

Tracking methodology:

- All patients who registered for the bariatric surgery program were checked to see if they had signed up for the online blog.

- At the initial registration point, potential patients were questioned about the factors that influenced them to consider having surgery at Genesis. Individuals who indicated that the blog was the primary factor were noted.

- Individuals who then actually had bariatric surgery were tracked relative to (a) their utilization of the blog and (b) revenues generated from the surgery.

Factor for new patients to the organization:

- New patients were individuals participating in the bariatric surgery program who had not used Genesis for care within the prior five years. The 80 patients coming from the blog all fit this criterion.

Factor for business they would have gotten anyway:

- The bariatric surgery program was considered to be more of a regional service and thus the organization opted to use the market share base for the Quad Cities area rather than the immediate Scott County primary service area. This market share level was 62%. Thus, for ROI purposes it was assumed that 62% of the bariatric surgery volume would have come to Genesis anyway.

In light of the relative newness of bariatric surgery at the time of this case, the use of a 62% factor for business they would have gotten anyway is probably overly conservative relative to the calculation of ROI.

Results/revenues/costs:

- Average charges per bariatric surgery case are approximately $30,000. The factor used for contractual allowances (which varies by payer) is 50%.

- The Genesis financial department opted to apply all costs—variable and fixed overhead—to this program. This very conservative approach to applying costs resulted in an average net revenue per case of $1,500 (again, net of contractuals, variable costs, and overhead costs).

- Using the factor for business they would have gotten anyway from above, the net cases attributed to the effort is 30 (38% of 80).

- Net revenues from the blog = 30 x $1,500 = $45,000

A Marketer's Guide to Measuring ROI

Calculation of effort ROI

$$\text{ROI\%} = \frac{\text{Net revenue} - \text{Marketing expense}}{\text{Marketing expense}} \times 100$$

$$\text{ROI\%} = \frac{(\$45,000 - \$19,500)}{\$19,500} \times 100$$

Effort ROI = 131%

 This is a very conservative effort ROI in light of the use of a market share level that is probably overstated for the program in question and the application of both variable and fixed overhead costs. Nonetheless, the model shows a positive effort ROI as a result of the bariatric surgery blog marketing program.

Case study 2: Covenant Medical Center

Sources

John Berg, director of business development at Covenant Medical Center, and Ann Theis, senior consultant at The Strategy Group.

Organizational background

Covenant Medical Center is a 650-bed provider organization that includes two acute care campuses, an inpatient physical rehabilitation facility, and nearly 20 outpatient locations. The organization is one of the largest healthcare providers in Michigan and serves a 15-county area in mid-Michigan. In any given year, Covenant sees more than 29,000 inpatient admissions and handles nearly 3,500 births. Competition comes from one other acute care organization in Saginaw and hospitals in two neighboring cities.

Program-marketing effort

In early 2005, Covenant introduced a new program to the local market called Women's Heart Advantage. These kinds of membership marketing programs are designed to position a hospital or healthcare organization as a leader in heart-related services for women in its local market and, through this positioning, capture a greater share of female cardiology care. Women's Heart Advantage is a turn-key program purchased from an external third party. The program was in place at more than 100 hospitals and health systems nationally prior to Covenant's introduction of the program into its local market. Enrollment in the program is free, and women who join receive the following benefits:

- A heart health kit including information on women's heart health issues, a bookmark, a pin, and other heart-related materials.

- A welcome call from the Center for the Heart (a Covenant clinical service line).

- A quarterly newsletter focusing on heart health issues for women.

- A free yearly heart health screening including a health risk appraisal, a cholesterol-related blood test, and a face-to-face review of the results with a program nurse. Members with borderline results are either referred back to their own physician (with results forwarded to the physician) or are referred to appropriate resources for further testing or treatment.

- Quarterly educational events.

- A guide to healthy fast-food choices and a heart-healthy cookbook.

Covenant introduced Women's Health Advantage in mid-January 2005 on a limited basis, targeting only employees of the hospital and staff of hospital-affiliated physician offices. This was done to give the organization some experience and to work out the kinks prior to communitywide launch. In February 2005, the program was opened up to women in the Covenant service area. Promotional efforts included public relations (media placements); community events; Web site coverage; direct mail; and paid advertising via outdoor, print, radio, and television outlets.

An initial attempt at effort ROI was conducted in May 2006, looking at the period of January through December 2005. Some relevant program statistics (as of December 2005):

- 3,500 women became members of the program (it had more than 9,000 members as of April 2007)

- 469 members participated in the free heart health screening

- Preference share for cardiology services among female consumers rose from 22% (pre–program launch) to 29%

ROI analysis information and assumptions

Marketing effort elements:
- Program acquisition
- Members benefits (e.g., materials, newsletter, and screenings)
- Web site coverage
- Community events
- Earned media story placements
- Paid media advertising and direct mail

Marketing costs:
- Covenant calculated a marketing cost of $286,000 for the period of January through December 2005. It should be noted that this cost included the cost of acquiring the Women's Heart Advantage program plus media advertising, events, and all screening efforts.

 A Marketer's Guide to Measuring ROI

Time period for tracking results:

- January 1, 2005 through December 31, 2005

Results considered coming from the marketing effort:

- It was determined that all clinical volume coming from members of the Women's Heart Advantage program would be counted toward the marketing effort, not just care that might be deemed to be heart-related.

- Part of this decision was driven by a presumption that the program and cardiology-related care has a halo impact on overall preference for and use of a specific provider.

- Part of the decision was also driven by the consideration that it was very challenging for Covenant to isolate cardiology-only usage. For example, a CT scan conducted for a heart-related purpose would show up as revenue in diagnostic imaging and not in the cardiology service line.

Tracking methodology:

- The tracking of results from the Women's Heart Advantage program looked at usage volumes coming from two categories of members: Overall hospital usage by members deemed to be new to Covenant and the differential in usage by nonnew members based on the average of the two 12-month periods prior to January 2005 versus the usage during the period of January through December 2005.

• The tracking process was significantly facilitated by the presence within the Covenant organization of a master patient information database. This database was created with support from an external vendor and covers patient activity from multiple sources including urgent care; occupational health; employed practices; and hospital inpatient, outpatient, and ER services. This database allows the organization to look at the specific activity and revenues generated by identifiable individuals.

Factor for new patients:

• A new patient was considered to be one who had not used Covenant Medical Center for any type of clinical care in the three-year period prior to the start of the program (i.e., after January 2002). Because this criterion was not rolled forward as the program progressed, the determination of a new patient eventually stretched to nearly four years.

• This was determined via an electronic record-reconciliation between the Women's Health Advantage membership roster and hospital medical records.

Factor for business would have gotten anyway:

• Because all usage (regardless of the clinical nature) by Women's Heart Advantage members was considered coming from the marketing effort, no factor for business that would have come anyway was implemented for this effort ROI. It should be noted that this was a deliberate determination by the Covenant Medical Center leadership, who felt that since the goal of a membership type of marketing program is to create a proactive relationship with consumers, the goal should be to develop loyalty and, by extension, increase utilization of services. As a result,

A Marketer's Guide to Measuring ROI

looking at new patients and gains from existing patients involved in the program was the appropriate approach.

Results/revenues/costs:

- Out of 3,504 Women's Heart Advantage members, 1,899 became patients at Covenant Medical Center by December 31, 2005.

- 90 of these patients were deemed to be new to Covenant. These 90 individuals generated 159 encounters and $65,261 in net patient revenues (collected).

- 1,809 of these patients were deemed not to be new to Covenant. These 1,809 individuals generated 10,512 encounters and $3,122,071 in net patient revenues. The average usage in the two years prior to the start of the Women's Health Advantage program was 1,303 patients, 8,173 encounters, and $2,751,342 in net patient revenues (all from the pool of Women's Heart Advantage members).

- As a result, the net patient revenue attributed to members of the Women's Heart Advantage program was $65,261 (from new members) plus $370,729 (the differential between the postprogram usage and the average of the two years prior to program start for all program members). Total net patient revenue was $65,261, plus $370,729, for a total of $435,990.

- The factor for direct costs (costs of services provided) was approximated at 50%. (Note: An estimate was used for the initial analysis for 2005 because the Covenant financial systems could not provide a specific level of direct costs by clinical service. According to Covenant representatives, system improvements will provide them with more exact cost percentages in 2007 and going forward).

- The net revenue from Women's Heart Advantage members after direct costs was $217,995 for the period of January to December 2005.

Calculation of effort ROI:

$$ROI\% = \frac{\text{Net revenue} - \text{Marketing expense}}{\text{Marketing expense}} \times 100$$

$$ROI\% = \frac{(\$217,995 - \$286,000}{\$286,000} \times 100$$

$$\text{Effort ROI} = -24\%$$

 A Marketer's Guide to Measuring ROI

On the surface, this is a negative effort ROI for the period of January 1, 2005 through December 31, 2005. Revenues generated from members of the program did not fully cover the marketing costs, even after the subtraction of the direct costs of providing care. However, the marketing costs are significantly front-end loaded. In other words, all of the costs of purchasing the program from the external vendor were included in this initial 12-month measurement, which impacted the short-term ROI. While information was not available at press time, measurements for the 12-month period of 2006 are expected to show a better effort ROI as membership grows, more new users are attracted, and the program acquisition costs are spread out over a longer period of time. This case is a good example of why marketing often needs to be considered an investment that requires time (and patience) to see to fruition.

Case study 3: Cleveland Clinic Foundation—orthopedics

Sources

Jim Blazar, chief marketing, communications, and new product development officer, and Sylvia Morrison, director of database marketing.

Organizational background

The Cleveland Clinic Foundation is an internationally recognized healthcare provider, research, and teaching organization. The foundation includes a 1,000-bed flagship hospital in Cleveland, a network of community hospitals in the metro Cleveland area, a full-service hospital and clinic site in Florida, a number of family healthcare and ambulatory surgery centers in the metro Cleveland area, and 1,600 salaried physicians in 120 specialties and sub-specialties.

As an organization, the Cleveland Clinic sees more than 2,800,000 outpatient visits and 70,000 inpatient admissions per year. Patients come to the Cleveland Clinic from all over the United States and from more than 80 different countries worldwide. *U.S. News & World Report* ranks it as one of the top three hospitals in the United States.

Marketing effort

In March 2006, the Cleveland Clinic conducted a public educational program for consumers about osteoarthritis. The program featured both medical and surgical specialists and focused on the nonsurgical and surgical (hip and knee replacement) options available to patients. The free program was held at one of the Cleveland Clinic's family health centers in the metro Cleveland area. Marketing support for this seminar included a single-mailing direct mail piece (postcard) aimed at consumers using specific medications or with specific self-identified conditions. A total of 5,000 qualified names were obtained via a purchased list. Targeted consumers had to be age 50 and over, have a household income in excess of $50,000, and live within 5–7 miles of the family health center. The mailing was sent to 4,750 people on the purchased list (with 250 or 5% held out as a control group). Interested consumers could register for the program via the call center or online.

ROI analysis information and assumptions

Marketing effort elements:
- Purchase of qualified mailing list
- Single-mailing postcard
- Educational seminar with Cleveland Clinic medical and surgical subspecialists

A Marketer's Guide to Measuring ROI

Marketing costs:

- $1,785 for the costs of printing, postage, and handling

Note: All material design work and production was done in-house and Cleveland Clinic's leadership decided not to include staff time as a marketing cost for ROI tracking purposes.

Time period for tracking results:

- Results were tracked for a period of one year from the date of the seminar (March 26, 2006)

Results considered coming from the marketing effort:

- To be counted as coming from this specific education seminar, patients had to utilize services related to orthopedic surgery (surgery, physician visits, MRI, physical therapy, etc.)

Tracking methodology:

- The Cleveland Clinic has a relational database for all consumers and households, which provides the organization with a detailed profile of utilization and revenues generated

- Participants from the seminar were tracked for 12 months after the event to examine if they utilized orthopedic-related services

Factor for new patients:

- New patients were deemed to be individuals who (a) attended the seminar and (b) did not have a Clinic ID number prior to the seminar. This meant that they had never used a Cleveland Clinic facility or physician for patient care prior to attending this program.

Factor for business would have gotten anyway:

- In light of the clear definition of a new patient, it was deemed unnecessary for this ROI analysis to also include a factor for business they would have gotten anyway.

Results/revenues/costs:

- 121 people attended the seminar (a 2.5% response rate based on a mailing of 4,750 people).

- 87 people who then came in for an orthopedic-related consult were deemed to be new (they did not have a Clinic ID number).

- 338 visits or encounters (MRI, doctor visit, physical therapy, etc.) were generated.

- 17 received orthopedic surgery.

- $104,715 in net revenues were generated after the application of direct and indirect costs. (Note: The clinic leadership determined that the ROI model to be used to track marketing efforts would include both direct and indirect costs.)

- The control group (250 names pulled from the original purchased list) generated no participation in the seminar and no new patients to Cleveland Clinic for orthopedic-related care during the evaluation period.

 A Marketer's Guide to Measuring ROI

Calculation of effort ROI

$$\text{ROI\%} = \frac{\text{Net revenue} - \text{Marketing expense}}{\text{Marketing expense}} \times 100$$

$$\text{ROI\%} = \frac{(\$104,\!715 - \$1,\!785)}{\$1,\!785} \times 100$$

Effort ROI = 5,766% (Note: The Cleveland Clinic uses a ratio model internally: 58 to 1)

As discussed above, the Clinic opts not to include the costs of marketing staff time in their ROI analyses. Based on informal input, the staff time to support this project was estimated to be equal to $15,000. If included it would result in an effort ROI of 530% or a ratio of 5.3 to 1.

Case study 4: Cleveland Clinic Foundation—pediatrics

Sources

Jim Blazar, chief marketing, communications, and new product development officer, and Sylvia Morrison, director of database marketing.

Organizational background

In addition to the resources and service lines noted in the previous case study, The Cleveland Clinic has had a formal Children's Hospital for 17 years. The primary competitor in the area (Rainbow Babies & Children's Hospital) has been established in the market for more than 100 years.

Marketing effort

In 2003, The Cleveland Clinic determined that 48% of the family physicians, pediatricians, and pediatric subspecialists in a designated service area (mostly Northeast Ohio) had made a referral for pediatric care during the prior year. The clinic routinely sent mailings to these physicians with information about its physicians, capabilities, etc. One of these mailings was a four-page quarterly newsletter. Each issue focused on a specific clinical case and the physician/clinical team supporting that case. This newsletter was produced internally (content, printing, etc.). The July 2006 issue of the pediatric newsletter focused on clinical cases involving rehabilitation and autism. The mailing was sent to 3,844 current and potential referral sources (family physicians, pediatricians, and pediatric specialists) in the designated geographic area.

ROI analysis information and assumptions

A Marketer's Guide to Measuring ROI

Marketing effort elements:

- Four-page pediatric newsletter sent to actual and potential referring physicians (family practice, pediatricians, and pediatric specialists) in a designated geographic area in Northeast Ohio

Marketing costs

- $1,230 for the costs of printing, postage, and handling

(Note: All material design work and production was done in-house and the leadership chose not to include staff time as a marketing cost for ROI tracking purposes.)

Time period for tracking results

- Referrals from the targeted physician pool were tracked from August 1, 2006 through March 31, 2007 (eighr months)

Results considered coming from the marketing effort

- Clinical cases had to involve the areas covered in the specific issue of the newsletter—rehabilitation or autism care

Tracking methodology

- The referral sources for all patients are tracked in the organization's relational database. This database tracks all usage and revenues by consumer and household.

- Clinic staff noted cases matching the clinical criteria coming from physicians who had never made a referral to the clinic for pediatric care prior to this mailing.

Factor for new patients:
- New patients were deemed to be individuals who (a) were referred by a physician who received the newsletter and who had never made a referral before and (b) did not have a Clinic ID number.

Factor for business would they have gotten anyway:
- Since the tracked volumes came from physicians who had never made a referral for pediatric care it was not deemed relevant to consider a factor for business they would have gotten anyway.

Results/revenues/costs:
- Fourteen targeted physicians who had never referred a pediatric case made a referral (for the related clinical conditions) after receiving this specific issue of the newsletter.

- These new referral sources sent 18 patients who generated 21 visits by the close of the tracking period. All of these patients were deemed to be new to the Cleveland Clinic.

- $2,482 in net revenues were generated after the application of direct and indirect costs. (Note: The clinic's leadership determined that the ROI model to be used to track marketing efforts would include both direct and indirect costs.)

Calculation of effort ROI:

$$\text{ROI\%} = \frac{\text{Net revenue} - \text{Marketing expense}}{\text{Marketing expense}} \times 100$$

$$\text{ROI\%} = \frac{(\$2{,}482 - \$1{,}230)}{\$1{,}230} \times 100$$

$$\text{Effort ROI} = 102\%$$

 This level of effort ROI is just above breakeven. However, the cases **Author's note** profiled in this particular issue of the newsletter, rehabilitation and autism, are not episodic in nature. Care for some of these patients is likely to continue for some time to come and thus there are almost certainly going to be downstream revenues that will improve the ROI picture. A measurement period of eight months may not be sufficient to show the impact of this specific marketing activity.

Case study 5: M. D. Anderson Cancer Center

Sources

Alicia Jansen, executive director of marketing, M. D. Anderson Cancer Center; and Victor Honadijy, program manager, strategic marketing, at M. D. Anderson Cancer Center.

Organizational background

The University of Texas M. D. Anderson Cancer Center in Houston is a well-regarded 518-bed facility devoted exclusively to cancer patient care, research, education, and prevention. It offers inpatient and outpatient care to more than 79,000 people from all over the world each year, including 27,000 new patients.

Marketing effort

In early 2006, the M. D. Anderson leadership decided to track financial ROI in two distinct markets in Texas with a paid media marketing effort. The two markets included in this effort were the Corpus Christi and the Beaumont MSA's. Both are reasonably close to the Houston area but neither market had ever been the focus of a concerted marketing effort by the organization, outside of the passive impact of general public relations, physician relations, or media placement efforts. The objectives of the marketing effort were to (a) increase the number of newly diagnosed cancer patients over historical levels coming from the two areas and (b) to influence the payer mix of patients coming from these two markets.

Marketing, PR, and physician relations at M. D. Anderson are distinct functions. In determining if Corpus Christi and Beaumont were appropriate

 A Marketer's Guide to Measuring ROI

markets for an ROI tracking effort, the organization's marketing function conferred with the PR and physician relations functions to determine if any active efforts had been going on or were planned for either MSA.

The development of the effort ROI tracking process at M. D. Anderson took place over a period of six months and involved meetings with the finance leadership and other key areas to determine the availability of data and the acceptability of the tracking methodology.

Because the organization only provides cancer-related care, the ability to determine acceptable results from a marketing effort is very straight-forward. Three categories of patients were considered as acceptable coming from this campaign—patients who are diagnosed by physicians in the target areas and referred to M. D. Anderson for care, patients who come to M. D. Anderson and are then diagnosed as having cancer by the M. D. Anderson staff, and patients who come to M. D. Anderson after being treated elsewhere.

ROI analysis information and assumptions

Marketing effort elements:

- Baseline market research.

- Print, radio and television advertising. This advertising included elements that could be considered to be both "brand" and demand generation" in scope.

Marketing costs:
- Costs include market research, media advertising design, and placement and allocated staff time. Beaumont's marketing costs were $96,213. Corpus Christi's marketing costs were $96,902.

Time period for tracking results:
- The marketing effort was initiated in March of 2006. Tracking of effort ROI is projected to go for two years (through March of 2008).

- Interim measurements will be conducted every six months.

- The effort ROI for this case is based on the period of March 2006 through August of 2006 (six months).

- Analysis was not completed until April of 2007 due to internal financial system issues related to being able to track volumes and associated revenues.

Tracking methodology:
- Due to the nature of the call center structure at M. D. Anderson (multiple call center functions by clinical area, not under the control of marketing) a "direct connect" approach was not practical.

- Because usage from the target markets had been relatively steady over time and no other extraneous events had occurred (such as a major PR effort by M. D. Anderson or the closure of a competing program) it was felt that looking at changes in volumes/revenues coming after the start of the marketing campaign would be a viable way to track the effort ROI.

- With the support of finance and other key areas, marketing examined patient volumes and revenues coming from Corpus Christi and Beaumont in fiscal year 2005 versus the tracking period of fiscal year 2006 (March 2006 through August of 2006).

Factor for new patients to the organization:
- Based on the nature of the clinical care provided by M. D. Anderson, all cases coming to the organization from the target markets were considered to be new. This included new patients served and newly diagnosed cancer cases.

Factor for business they would have gotten anyway:
- Business that the organization would have gotten anyway was considered to be the baseline level from 2005. Any changes beyond that level were considered to be new business and were counted as coming from the marketing effort.

Results/revenues/costs:
- Patient volumes increased by 19% from the Beaumont area and 10% from the Corpus Christi area during the initial six month tracking period (over the same six month period from prior to the campaign).

- Beaumont had 1,140 cases in fiscal year 2006, up from 959 in the previous fiscal year.

- Corpus Christi had 372 cases in fiscal year 2006, up from 338 in the previous fiscal year.

- There were also positive shifts in payer mix towards Blue Cross and PPO plans.

- Working with the M. D. Anderson finance department, it was determined that the effort ROI model needed to include (a) patient revenues defined as actual payments received for care and (b) all variable costs—both direct and indirect.

- Net revenues gained (total payments less all variable costs): $203,599 for Beaumont and $1,755,853 for Corpus Christi. (The differential in net revenues by target market is partially explained by the complexity of the oncology cases that were received from the different markets.)

 A Marketer's Guide to Measuring ROI

Calculation of effort ROI:

$$\text{ROI\%} = \frac{\text{Net revenue} - \text{Marketing expense}}{\text{Marketing expense}} \times 100$$

$$\text{Beaumont ROI} = \frac{\$203,599 - \$96,213}{\$96,213} \times 100$$

Beaumont effort ROI = 112%

$$\text{Corpus Christi ROI} = \frac{\$1,755,853 - \$96,902}{\$96,902} \times 100$$

Corpus Christi ROI = 1,712%

Author's note

The M. D. Anderson marketing staff anticipate that the effort ROI results from Beaumont and Corpus Christi will change and even out during the course of the two year marketing and results tracking effort. The high ROI for the Corpus Christi effort reflects the clinical mix of cases received during the initial six month time period.